Elbow Arthroscopy and Minimal Invasive Surgery

Andreas B. Imhoff • Andreas Lenich
Editors

Elbow Arthroscopy and Minimal Invasive Surgery

Edited and Translated by Hani Eltair

Springer

Editors

Andreas B. Imhoff
Department of Orthopaedic Sports Medicine
Rechts der Isar Hospital
München, Germany

Andreas Lenich
Department for Trauma and Orthopaedic Surgery
Josephinum Klinikum
München, Germany

ISBN 978-3-031-75610-8 ISBN 978-3-031-75611-5 (eBook)
https://doi.org/10.1007/978-3-031-75611-5

Previous editions published with Springer-Verlag Berlin Heidelberg

Based on the translation from the German language edition: "Arthroskopie und minimal-invasive Chirurgie des Ellenbogens" by Andreas B. Imhoff and Andreas Lenich, © Springer-Verlag GmbH Deutschland, ein Teil von Springer Nature 2018. Published by Springer Berlin, Heidelberg. All Rights Reserved.

This Springer imprint is published by the registered company Springer Nature Switzerland AG
The registered company address is: Gewerbestrasse 11, 6330 Cham, Switzerland

Preface

In just a few years, arthroscopy of the elbow has become a remarkable tool in the treatment of elbow disorders. These advanced surgical techniques enable precise diagnosis and treatment of elbow pathologies while minimizing soft tissue irritation. Minimally invasive techniques offer patients less invasive treatment options, potentially resulting in reduced recovery times.

The unique anatomical structure of the elbow joint, with its compact spaces and proximity to critical neurovascular structures, has historically posed challenges to surgeons. However, advances in surgical instrumentation, imaging technologies, and procedural techniques have enabled surgeons to overcome these obstacles. These innovations facilitate precise diagnostic and therapeutic interventions, minimize surgical trauma, accelerate recovery, and optimize clinical outcomes for patients.

This book provides a comprehensive and practical resource for both seasoned surgeons and those new to elbow arthroscopy and minimally invasive approaches. By highlighting key techniques and potential pitfalls, this guide helps readers to master these complex procedures while prioritizing patient safety and achieving surgical excellence.

München, Germany — Andreas Lenich
München, Germany — Andreas B. Imhoff

Contents

Abbreviations

AO	Working group for osteosynthesis issues (Arbeitsgemeinschaft für Osteosynthesefragen)
aMCL	Anterior bundle of the medial collateral ligament
a.p.	Anterior posterior
ASK	Arthroscopy
ASSH	American Society for Surgery of the Hand
C	Cervical
CEO	Common extensor origin
CPM	Continuous passive motion
CRAP	Classification system for the lateral elbow pain
CRPS	Complex regional pain syndrome
D	Digits
ECRB	Extensor carpi radialis brevis
EHR	Epicondylitis humeri radialis (lateral epicondylitis)
Ext.	Extension
FJB	Free joint loose body
Flex.	Flexion
G	Gauge
HO	Heterotopic ossification
IR	Implant removal
K-wire	Kirschner wire
Lig.	Ligament
LCL	Lateral collateral ligament
LUCL	Lateral ulnar collateral Ligament
M./Mm.	Muscle/Muscles
MACT	Matrix-induced autologous cartilage cell transplantation
MCL	Medial collateral ligament
MMP	Matrix metalloproteinases
MUCL	Medial ulnar collateral ligament
N./Nn.	Nerve/Nerves
OATS	Osteochondral autograft transfer system
OCA	Osteocapsular arthroplasty
OCL	Osteochondral lesion
OD	Osteochondritis dissecans
PAP	Preoperative antibiotic prophylaxes
PIN	Posterior interosseous nerve (radial nerve, innervates the forearm extensors)

PLRI	Posterolateral rotational instability
pMCL	Posterior bundle of the medial collateral ligament
PRUJ	Proximal radioulnar joint
ROM	Range of motion
TEP	Total endoprosthesis (arthroplasty)
UA	Upper arm
V./Vv.	Vein/Veins

Anatomy and Biomechanics of the Elbow Joint

1

K. Wegmann, M. Hackl, and L. P. Müller

Contents

1.1 Introduction

The elbow is not an isolated articulated structure. The functional connection with the forearm and also the wrist should be considered while studying the elbow. Native biomechanics and pathobiomechanics are inextricably linked. As in all joints of the human body, the functionality of the elbow joint is based on a balanced interplay between mobility and stability. In the following, the anatomical and biomechanical basics around the elbow will be conveyed. These form the basics for understanding, recognizing, and treating various elbow pathologies. It is essential to know the relative contributions of the individual joint stabilizers to adequately treat dislocation fractures.

The anatomy and biomechanics of the elbow joint are discussed below according to their functional unit.

K. Wegmann
OCM (Orthopädische Chirurgie München) Clinic, München, Germany
e-mail: kilian.wegmann@ocm-muenchen.de

M. Hackl · L. P. Müller (✉)
Department of Orthopedic and Trauma Surgery, University Hospital Cologne, Cologne, Germany
e-mail: michael.hackl@uk-koeln.de; lars.mueller@uk-koeln.de

A. B. Imhoff, A. Lenich (eds.), *Elbow Arthroscopy and Minimal Invasive Surgery*,
https://doi.org/10.1007/978-3-031-75611-5_1

1.2 Distal Humerus

The bony structure gives the elbow a characteristic configuration (Fig. 1.1). The frontal view is dominated by the medial and lateral epicondyle, which emerges from the humeral shaft via the supracondylar crest and serves as the origin for the flexors and extensors and through their prominent position they lengthen their lever arm. In rare cases, there is a rudimentary supracondylar process proximal to the medial epicondyle, which can be the cause of neurovascular compression syndromes. If you connect the medial and the lateral epicondyle by means of an imaginary line, the joint line is about 2 cm distal from this line. This information can be helpful during clinical examinations and also when creating incisions or arthroscopic portals. The joint-forming part of the distal humerus is in relation to the humeral shaft about 6–8° valgus and 5–6° internally rotated (Fig. 1.1). The joint block itself is flexed anteriorly by 29–31° in relation to the longitudinal axis of the humerus.

This characteristic configuration is based on the functional requirements. The valgus component of the forearm facilitates the precise axis rotation of the forearm, while the anterior flexion of the joint block serves as an offset and increases the ability of the elbow flexion. Deviations from the bony configuration of the distal humerus, for example, due to malunited fractures, lead to significant functional restrictions of the elbow joint and thus the entire forearm.

The dorsal deepening of the distal humerus and the olecranon fossa serves to receive the tip of the olecranon in extension and that guarantees the full extension through their shape, and this also ensures stability. The olecranon fossa is separated anteriorly from the radial and coronoid fossae by a bony membrane. The resulting spaces are filled with fatty tissue. If these fossae are filled with blood for example after fracture, the fluid level can be identified as a so-called "fat pad sign" in the X-ray.

The blood supply of the distal humerus is via a central artery that arises from the brachial artery. On the other hand, it is also supplied from recurrent ascending vessels that enter the distal humerus both laterally and medially. There is a special situation with regard to the lateral epicon-

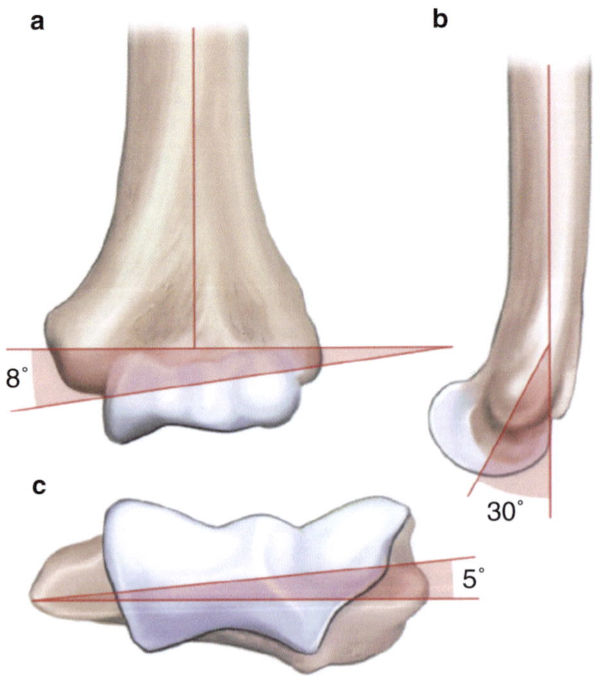

Fig. 1.1 Relationship of the articular surface to the humeral shaft. (**a**) In the frontal plane, the articular block is inclined 6–8° radially. (**b**) In the sagittal plane, the joint block is flexed anteriorly by about 30°. (**c**) In the transverse plane, the joint block shows a medial rotation between 3° and 6° (modified By Wegmann and Müller [19])

dyle, as the vessels mainly enter from the dorsal side [1]. In the area between the draining central vessel in the shaft and the distal, recurrent vessels, there is a watershed, with an increased risk of undersupply [2].

1.3 Medial Column

On the ulnar side, the articulation between the trochlea and the proximal ulna takes place. The trochlea is curved in a characteristic way like a coil and shows a high degree of conformity to the trochlear notch. The trochlea is covered with cartilage. On the ventral part of the trochlea, the cartilage is about 1.3 mm thick, in the dorsal area of the trochlea is about 0.8 mm [3] (Fig. 1.2). The high degree of accuracy of fit of the native humeroulnar joint results in an almost perfect or idealized hinge joint. There is no clearly defined axis of rotation in the elbow. As biomechanical studies have shown, there is a wandering center of rotation. In the sagittal plane, the center of rotation moves over an area of 7.8 × 2.5 mm [4], depending on the extension/flexion position of the joint. In contrast to this, the common models of dynamic elbow fixators and dynamic orthotics impose a rigid center of rotation on the joint. These measures undoubtedly represent sensible therapy tools.

The medial epicondyle serves as the origin of the medial collateral ligament apparatus. The anterior bundle of the medial collateral ligament, which represents the primary valgus stabilizer of the elbow, arises just above the center of rotation on the medial epicondylus [5] (Fig. 1.3). The joint capsule arises ventral or caudal to the ligament. The flexor group with the flexor carpis radialis muscle, the flexor carpi ulnaris muscle, and the flexor digitorum superficialis muscle originate cranially from the ligament. The pronator teres muscle arises proximally to this group at the upper edge of the medial epicondyle [6].

The anterior bundle of the medial collateral ligament in 90° flexion makes the greatest contribution to the valgus stability of the elbow. Functionally, the anterior bundle is divided into an anterior and a posterior part. The anterior part relaxes in flexion and tenses in extension (Fig. 1.4). The dorsal ligament behaves in the opposite way, and the anterior bundle of the medial collateral ligament shows a reciprocal behavior. Since the ligament does not originate directly from the center of rotation and has a

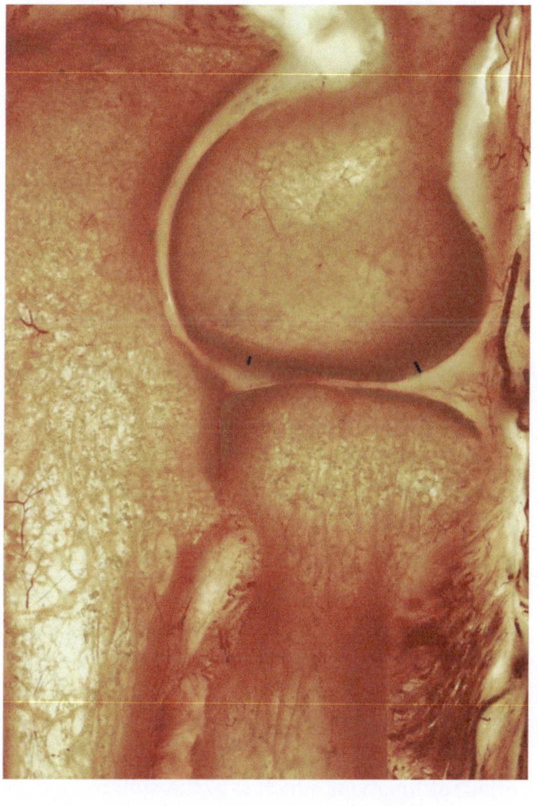

Fig. 1.2 Presentation of the cartilage thickness (black lines) decreasing from ventral to dorsal capitulum

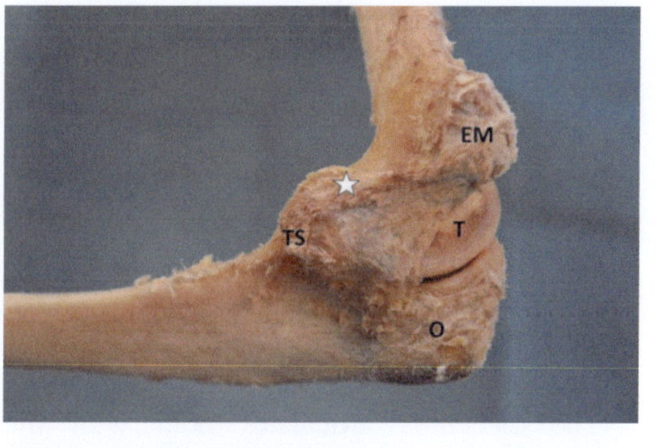

Fig. 1.3 Medial collateral ligament. *EM* Medial epicondyle, *TS* sublime tubercle, *T* trochlea, *O* olecranon, *Star*: anterior bundle of the medial collateral ligament

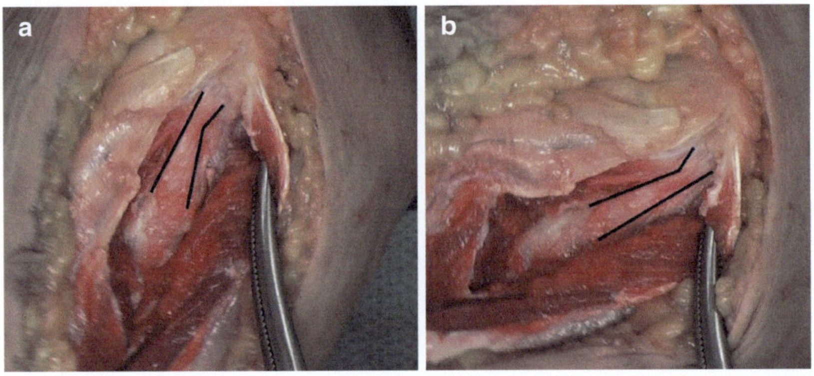

Fig. 1.4 Reciprocal behavior of the anterior bundle of the medial collateral ligament. (**a**) In extension, the anterior portion of the ligament is taut, and the dorsal portion is lax. (**b**) Conversely, in flexion, the dorsal part is tensed, and the anterior part is lax

reciprocal behavior, the medial ligament is not to be considered as an isometric ligament. The anterior bundle inserts into the sublime tubercle of the proximal ulna. Proximally and in the middle, the band is about 6 mm wide, and the insertion on the ulna is then widened to 9 mm [7]. In the case of the average stressed collateral ligament, a physiological thickening compared to the less stressed opposite side was demonstrated [7].

In the lateral view of the elbow, the tip of the olecranon plunges into the olecranon fossa of the distal humerus in extension and represents an important stabilizing function. Biomechanical studies have shown that resection of the tip of the olecranon of more than 25% leads to significant valgus instability [8].

The tip of the olecranon follows a characteristic concave curve distally, which ends in the coronoid process. In the sagittal plane, this results in a crescent form into which the distal humerus and the trochlea fit together. The opening angle of this crescent measures around 182° [9]. The high degree of conformity of the two structures offers an excellent fit and thus tight guidance. Conversely, however, this conformity must also be observed for fracture reduction. Thus, the reconstruction of the alignment of the dorsal cortex of the proximal ulna is recommended here and not the adaptation of the cartilage-bearing parts of the semi-lunar incisura. Otherwise, there is a risk of closing the trochlear notch and thus generating a limitation of movements.

The olecranon articulates both with the humerus via the trochlear notch and the radial head via the radial notch. A physiological "bare area" with an average length of 5 mm appears in the trochlear notch (Fig. 1.5a). There is little mechanical stimulation in this area since there is physiologically no contact with the humerus, and therefore no cartilage is developed [4]. In the fracture situation, this area must not be misinterpreted as a debris zone to be reconstructed to adapt the cartilage surface together.

The olecranon is characterized by a high individual anatomical variance. The ulnar shaft has a radially closed angle of 17–18°, which is known as the "radial bow" (Fig. 1.5). In addition, there is ventral angulation—the dorsal cranial cortex is convex—about 6° [10] (Fig. 1.6). If this dorsal angulation is under or over corrected in case of fracture treatment, an extension or flexion deficit will eventually result in the elbow joint. The high anatomical variance must be taken into account when choosing the osteosynthesis material.

The distal extension of the trochlear notch ends in the coronoid process. This hook-shaped extension completes the olecranon to form a crescent-shaped shape and helps to compensate for anteroposterior forces on the elbow. The average height of the coronoid is just below 17 mm [11]. On the coronoid process, the tip, the anteromedial facet, and the sublime tubercle can be distinguished. The anteromedial facet serves as a varus stabilizer so that it acts as a resistance to the medial trochlea under varus load [12].

The anteromedial facet bulges out on the medial ulna metaphysis, thus expanding the articular surface. The anterior bundle of the medial collateral ligament attaches to the sublime tubercle, which is medial to the anteromedial facet. If

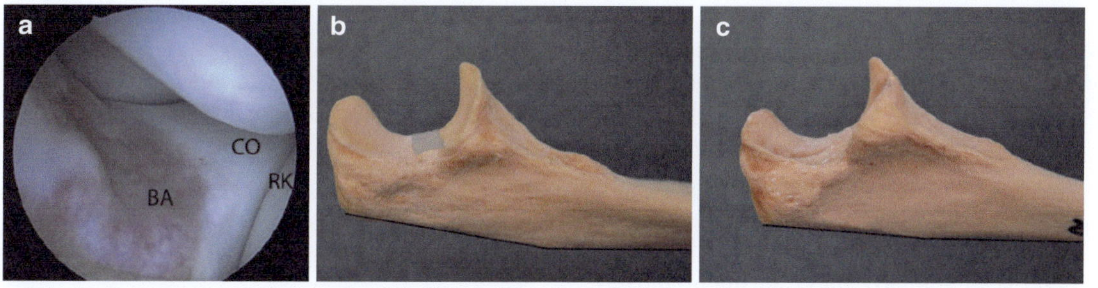

Fig. 1.5 (**a**) Bare area (BA) in the articular surface of the proximal ulna. (CO) coronoid process, (RK) radial head. (**b**, **c**) Interindividual variance of the dorsal angulation of the proximal ulna

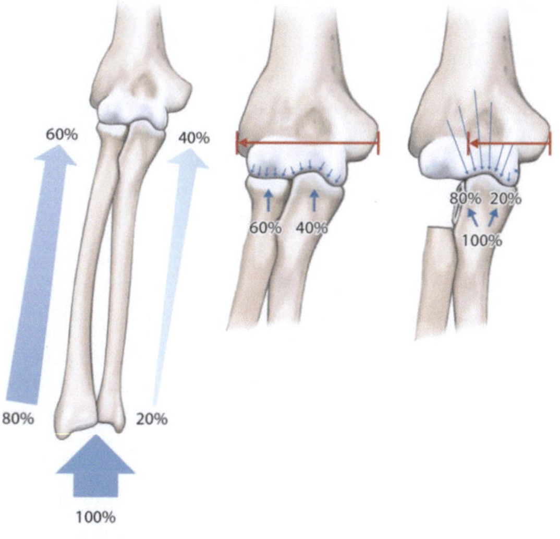

Fig. 1.6 Schematic presentation of the longitudinal force transmission in the forearm. When the forearm is intact, after approximately 80° of the applied load has been absorbed over the distal radius, it is redistributed through the interosseous membrane to the ulna. At the elbow, about 60% of the force hits the capitulum and 40% hits the trochlea. In case of a defect in the radius head, e.g., after resection of the radius head, the entire force is transferred to the medial column (modified by Wegmann and Müller [19])

the ligament is structurally intact, fractures that affect this area of the ulna can lead to failure of the medial ligament and consequent instability.

In addition to the anteroposterior stabilization, the coronoid was also identified as an important varus stabilizer [13]. To a small extent, it also contributes to the valgus stability. The brachialis muscle inserts about 10 mm distal to the coronoid tip. The joint capsule attaches about 2 mm to the coronoid tip [11]. The majority of the coronoid process is to be considered as a free-standing protrusion, which accordingly has little solid bony support. It is therefore not surprising that the coronoid process is often affected by injuries.

There is variable information about the need for refixation of the coronoid tip fractures to restore the integrity of the anterior joint capsule. In a small case series, a positive stabilization effect after the refixation of coronoid tip fractures was reported [14].

1.4 Lateral Column

The lateral part of the articular surface of the distal humerus, the capitulum, articulates with the radius head. Here, the conformity of the two structures has an important functional significance. The convex capitulum allows the concave radius head to rotate freely. However, sliding during the extension/flexion movements is also possible. The cartilage thickness at the capitulum is between 1.49 and 1.63 mm anteriorly and between 0.87 and 1.06 mm posteriorly [3]. However, this fitting also enables translational stability. A recent biomechanical study by Irish and colleagues underlines the relevance of the depression in the center of the radial head based on the nature of radial head prostheses [15]. It has been shown that the contact area and the contact pressure between the capitulum and the radial head depend on the depth of the articular surface of the radial head. The lowest pressure and the largest contact area were found at 3.2 ± 0.7 mm depth in the center of the radius head. The radius head is not round, but ellipsoid [16]. If the radius head is viewed in the neutral position of the forearm, a lateral enlargement is observed, which is the cause of its ellipsoidal shape. In pronation, the ellipsoidal shape appears to increase the frictional connection in the proximal radioulnar joint. According to anthropological research, this stabilization supported the precursors of the hominid primates during 4-legged gait with a pronated forearm [17]. In modern humans, the radial head similarly plays an important role in the axial stabilization of the forearm [18]. Biomechanical studies have shown that the radial column transfers 60% of the forces transmitted from the forearm to the distal humerus. At the wrist, the distal radius takes 80% of the load. The load is distributed via the interosseous membrane, which with its ascending and descending fibers influences the forces between the ulna and the radius [19, 20] (Fig. 1.6). This connection between the elbow, forearm, and wrist illustrates the close biomechanical connection of the structures and suggests that the individual areas in the trauma situation should not be viewed and treated separately but as a whole.

If the radial head is resected, 100% of the force acting on the forearm in the longitudinal direction passes through the medial column, which can lead to rapid degeneration of the corresponding articular cartilage. In addition, after resection of the radial head, valgus instability of the joint is not infrequently observed. After the anterior bundle of the medial collateral ligament, the radial head is considered as an important valgus stabilizer of the elbow [21]. Removing the radial head also has measurable consequences distal to the elbow joint. Lanting et al. demonstrated a significant increase in tension in the interosseous membrane of the forearm, which was reversible with a prosthetic radial head replacement [22]. In addition to the capitulum, the radial head articulates with the radial notch in the proximal radioulnar joint and with the lateral trochlear ridge. To ensure this articulation, the edge of the radial head is covered by 240° with cartilage, in the area in which it is in contact with the radial notch. The remaining 120° are only covered with cartilage on the narrow edge (articulation with the annular ligament (Fig. 1.7).

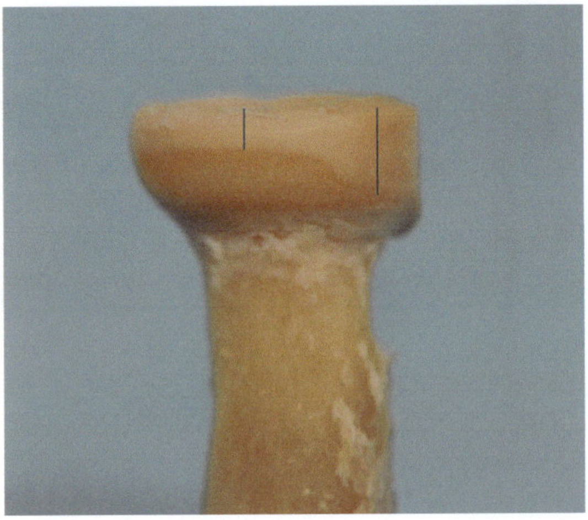

Fig. 1.7 Collar of the radius head. The area with a narrow band of cartilage cover represents the area that does not articulate with the proximal radioulnar joint (PRUG). The area with the broad cartilage ligament articulates with the incisura radialis ulnae (radial notch) in the PRUG

Correspondingly, the annular ligament contains cartilage partially on its inner side [23]. The annular ligament extends from the anterior border of the radial notch around the head of the radius to the dorsal border of the notch. In the context of osteosynthesis, a plate or prominent screw heads can be tolerated in the area of this 120° since no conflict with the proximal ulna is expected. The average diameter of the radial head is 22 mm, and the neck is angled 10–12°. Most of the available radius head prostheses do not yet allow these values to be reconstructed. In addition, it is not possible to reconstruct the articulation in the proximal radioulnar joint with conventional radius head prosthesis. The entire contact surface and the kinematics of the proximal radius are negatively influenced by the prosthesis implantation [24].

In addition to the bony fit, the lateral collateral ligament complex plays an important role in stabilizing the elbow joint. The lateral ligament complex consists of the annular ligament, the radial collateral ligament, the lateral ulnar collateral ligament, and the accessory radial collateral ligament (Fig. 1.8). The annular ligament stabilizes the radial head in the proximal radioulnar joint. In the future, it will be necessary to investi-

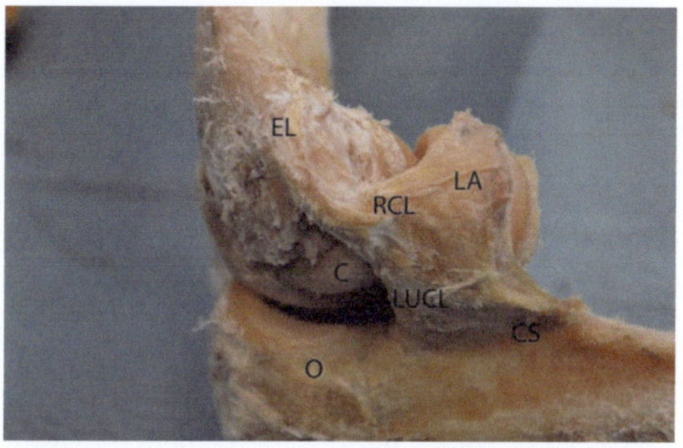

Fig. 1.8 Presentation of the lateral collateral ligament complex. *EL* lateral epicondyle, *RCL* radial collateral ligament, *LA* annular ligament, *C* capitulum, *LUCL* lateral ulnar collateral ligament, *CS* supinator crest

gate to what extent instabilities in the proximal radioulnar joint are clinically relevant and whether appropriate therapeutic measures are indicated.

The radial collateral ligament arises near the idealized center of rotation on the capitulum, extends distally on the joint capsule, and fuses with the annular ligament. It runs over the lateral edge of the radial head. An isometry has been demonstrated for the radial collateral band [25]. However, this is not the case with the lateral ulnar collateral ligament. It also arises near the idealized center of rotation on the capitulum and then extends to the supinator crest of the proximal ulna. It inserts together with the annular ligament on the proximal ulna. In the course of extension to flexion, the ligament experiences a relevant change in length with tension and increasing flexion, as Moritomo and colleagues were able to demonstrate [25].

The lateral ulnar collateral ligament is clearly not an isometric ligament. It pulls past the dorsolateral section of the radial head and thus functions like a hammock in which the radial head is stabilized. In addition, the ligament connects the ulna with the lateral epicondyle. A defect in the lateral collateral ligament can therefore lead to posterolateral rotational instability [26]. Here, the forearm rotates dorsally and laterally away from the distal humerus. This pathology was reported in particular by O'Driscoll and colleagues [27] and is explained in more detail in the following chapters (Chaps. 5 and 6). There are close anatomical relationships between the lateral ulnar collateral ligament, the posterolateral section of the radial head, and the joint capsule [28]. During arthroscopic debridement in the posterolateral joint section, iatrogenic damage to the ligament is possible.

1.5 Joint Capsule

The elbow joint, like the rest of the joints in the human body, is enclosed in a tight joint capsule. The different joint parts of the elbow are encompassed by this common capsule. There is a synovial layer on the joint side of the capsule. The capsule arises on the humerus shaft just proximal to the olecranon, radial, and coronoid fossae. The capsule inserts dorsally at the level of the annular ligament. The capsule inserts anteriorly, just distal to the coronoid tip on the medial side, and laterally it merges again into the annular ligament. Through the transition into the annular ligament, the joint capsule allows the radius to rotate freely. In the case of posttraumatic adhesions, the rotation of the radius can be compromised. Since the capsule surrounds the joint circumferentially, it plays an important role in the development of pathologies.

Instabilities and also joint stiffness can result from injuries to the joint capsule. The capsule has a filling volume, which is between 20 and 25 mL in the native joint, at around 80° of flexion. In the case of joints with capsular stiffness, the maximum filling volume can be reached even with significantly lower volumes.

1.6 Neuroanatomy

In terms of anatomy, there is a special situation at the elbow joint. The joint is crossed anteriorly and posteriorly as well as medially and laterally by important peripheral nerves. In almost every surgical procedure, the surgeon is confronted with the critical neural structures. A precise knowledge of neuroanatomy is essential to avoid serious complications. The literature offers a

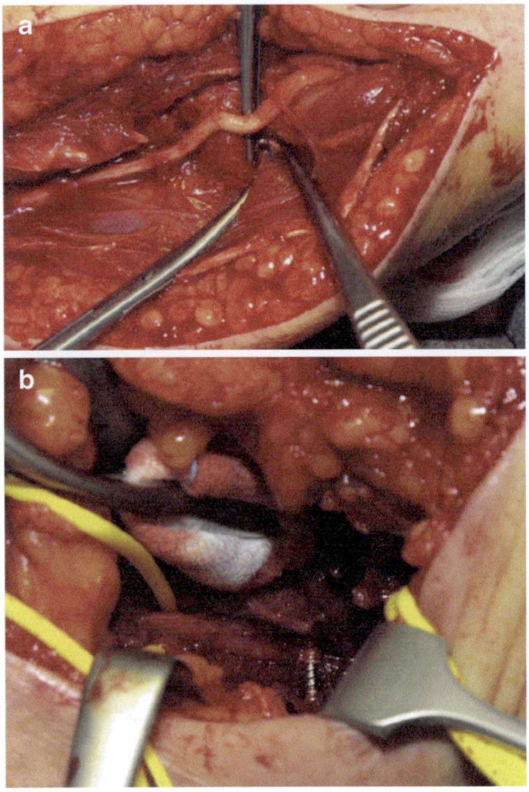

Fig. 1.9 (**a**) Position of the external fixator pins in relation to the ulnar nerve, approx. 10 cm proximal to the ulnar styloid process. (**b**) Illustration of the compression of the radial nerve on the lateral upper arm by a fixator pin. The nerve is marked by a yellow vessel loop

variety of case presentations that describe the corresponding iatrogenic nerve damage. In one case, the median and radial nerves were even severed during an arthroscopic operation [29]. The authors of this chapter have had the previously unpublished case of a 67-year-old patient in whom the ulnar and radial nerves were injured when an external fixator was applied to the elbow after a complex dislocation (Fig. 1.9). In some existing case series, the iatrogenic nerve damage is considered as the most common complication of elbow arthroscopy [30, 31].

1.6.1 Radial Nerve

The radial nerve and the median nerve are located anterior to the joint. The biceps tendon divides the soft tissues anterior to the joint into a medial and a lateral area. The radial nerve, which arises from the C5-Th1 segments, emerges from the posterior fasciculus of the brachial plexus. Below the clavicle, the nerve swings around the humeral shaft and then emerges in a spiral groove laterally in the radial sulcus. There it passes through the lateral intermuscular septum and then runs on the brachialis and medial and deep to the brachioradialis distally. At the level of the joint, the radial nerve can be found anterior to the medial margin of the capitulum. There it lies separated from the joint capsule by the belly of the brachialis muscle [32, 33]. When the elbow is fully extended, the nerve lies on average 10.8 mm medial to the lateral boundary of the capitulum and 5.5 mm anterior to it [32]. In 90° flexion, the nerve migrates 3.6 mm medially to lie approximately 14.4 mm medial to the lateral border of the capitulum. Additional insufflation of the joint with 20 mL of saline solution—as is done in arthroscopy—increases the distance to an average of 15.1 mm. The ventral distance increases to 10.8 mm in flexion, and the filling of the joint increases the distance to 17.0 mm.

However, the brachialis muscle is not always found distal to the joint line between the nerve and the joint capsule. This is especially important in arthroscopic procedures in which the joint capsule is resected. The risk of iatrogenic injury to the radial nerve is consequently increased distal to the joint line and laterally. Proximal to the joint at the level of the lateral epicondyle, it is divided into the superficial and the deep branches. The superficial branch runs distally under the brachioradialis muscle, for sensory supply of the the skin of the distal radial forearm and over the radial hand. Almost 10 cm proximal to the radial styloid process, the nerve emerges subcutaneously and supplies digitus (D I) radially and dorsally, and D II dorsally (sensory supply). The deep branch pushes deep and winds between the deep and superficial belly of the supinator muscle around the radial shaft in a dorsolateral direction. The ramus profundus (deep branch of the radial nerve) shows a position dependency with the rotational position of the forearm [34]. In supination, the nerve moves laterally with the supinator muscle; in pronation, the nerve moves medially. It is therefore advisable when performing a surgical intervention on the proximal radius, to be done from the lateral or posterolateral side, with the forearm in maximum pronation. This increases the distance between the ramus profundus and the radial head [34], which increases the safety of the respective surgical procedure.

1.6.2 Median Nerve

The median nerve runs medial to the biceps tendon and also arises from the C5-Th1 segments. It arises from the medial and lateral fasciculi of the brachial plexus; after it passes through the axilla, the median nerve runs anterior to the medial intermuscular septum in a distal direction. The nerve runs medial and deep to the brachial artery and its accompanying veins just proximal to the joint line. At the level of the joint line, in extension of the joint, the nerve runs an average of 5.9 mm lateral to the medial border of the trochlea and 4.8 mm anterior to it [32–34]. When flexed, the nerve moves 1.3 mm medially, with additional joint insufflation by 2.5–3.4 mm lateral to the medial delimitation of the trochlea. The distance to the ventral delimitation of the trochlea increases in 90° flexion to 8.4 mm, with additional insufflation the distance increases to 13.4 mm. The median nerve finally breaks through the pronator teres muscle and from there extends distally into the forearm. The guiding muscles for the forearm are the flexor digitorum superficialis and flexor digitorum profundus. The sensory fibers of the median nerve supply the radial part of the palm and the fingers I–III on the palmar side, as well as the radial half of the D-IV.

1.6.3 Ulnar Nerve

The third important peripheral nerve, the ulnar nerve runs past the elbow into the forearm and hand to provide critical sensory and motor functions. The ulnar nerve arises from the C8-Th1 segments from the medial fasciculus. The nerve runs in the medial bicipital sulcus anterior to the medial intermuscular septum. Approximately 10–12 cm proximal to the medial epicondyle, the ulnar nerve passes through the intermuscular septum and then enters the ulnar groove dorsal to the septum at the medial edge of the triceps [35]. The ulnar nerve lies superficially in the ulnar groove and is therefore exposed to mechanical irritation. In deep flexion, the nerve in the sulcus is stretched. The so-called Struthers Arcade [36] (Fig. 1.10) is often found proximal to the passage through the septum. It provides a connection between the medial septum and the fascia of the medial triceps head and can lead to ulnar nerve compression syndrome. Distal to the ulnar groove, the nerve pushes between the humeral and ulnar heads of the flexor carpi ulnaris muscle. At the joint level, the first motor branch of the ulnar nerve splits off, which initially runs with the nerve and then innervates the flexor carpi ulnaris muscle. Proximal to this, the ulnar nerve

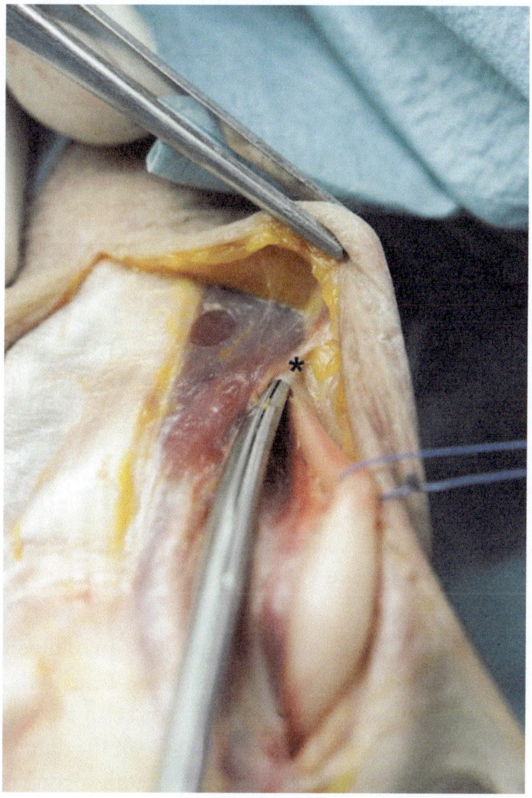

Fig. 1.10 *Star*: to the left of it, you can see the medial triceps head

only gives off sensory branches. The ulnar and humeral heads of the flexor carpi ulnaris muscle are connected by a connective tissue membrane that extends from the medial epicondyle to the olecranon. This is known as the Osborne Arcade [37]. Here, too, a compression syndrome of the ulnar nerve can occur if it is mechanically irritated during passage through the arcade. In the course of neurolysis of the ulnar nerve, it is important to explore and release these potential compression sites. This becomes even more important for ulnar nerve transposition since a transposition of the ulnar nerve with intact arcades leads to “kinking” of the nerves on the respective structures.

1.7 Muscles

Active mobility in the elbow joint is guaranteed by the muscles. The brachioradialis, brachialis, extensor carpi radialis, and biceps brachii are the flexors of the elbow joint. On the side of the extensors, the triceps brachii dominates, with a contribution from the flexor carpi ulnaris and anconeus. A valgus moment is caused by the extensor carpi ulnaris, the extensor carpi radialis, the extensor digitorum communis, and the brachioradialis muscles. A force in the sense of a varus load, however, is exerted by the flexor carpi radialis, the flexor digitorum (superficial and deeper parts), and the flexor carpi ulnaris. The strongest muscles on the flexor and extensor side are the brachialis and triceps brachii muscles, respectively.

The triceps brachii muscle shapes the dorsal aspect of the upper arm. It is innervated by the radial nerve and inserts into the olecranon with a strong tendon. The tendon does not only insert at the tip of the olecranon but merges flatly into the forearm fascia on the proximal ulna. On the radial side, the triceps brachii merges into the anconeus.

Medially it protects the ulnar nerve. If the medial head of the triceps is hypertrophic, or if there is another predisposition, the muscle belly may snap with symptoms similar to neuritis of the ulnar nerve or even be accompanied by irritation of the ulnar nerve.

The anconeus runs as a triangular muscle from the lateral epicondyle to the dorsolateral ulnar edge. Its direction is thus similar to that of the lateral ulnar collateral ligament. Since it presses the ulna to the lateral epicondyle through contraction and is thus similar to the holding function of the lateral ulnar collateral ligament, the muscle has already been referred to as an “active ligament” [38]. The specific role in elbow stability has not yet been clarified. As part of the embryonic development, the anconeus emerges from the medial triceps head in a distal direction and takes the innervation with it from there. Due to its origin on the upper arm, the anconeus is not a “real” forearm muscle. An indication of this is the strong fascia and a layer of fatty tissue that separates it from the directly adjacent extensor carpi ulnaris muscle and thus serves as a “pathway” during surgical interventions on the lateral elbow (Kocher interval). The anconeus muscle functions primarily as an extensor, but beyond 80° of flexion, it acts as a flexor [39]. On the ventral aspect of the upper arm, the biceps brachii dominate. The two-headed muscle arises from the supraglenoid tubercle and the coracoid process and inserts in the cubital fossa on the radial tuberosity. The innervation is provided by the musculocutaneous nerve. Functionally, the biceps brachii muscle is crucial in supination. The supinator muscle, which is responsible for the external rotation of the forearm, only plays a subordinate role here. The biceps brachii muscle is connected to the forearm fascia via the bicipital aponeurosis. When palpating the distal biceps tendon if structural damage is suspected, the bicipital aponeurosis can be mistaken for an intact biceps tendon. At the lateral edge of the distal biceps tendon the lateral cutaneous antebrachial nerve runs, which is the functional terminal branch of the musculocutaneous nerve. The brachialis muscle, which runs deep to the biceps brachii and is also innervated by the musculocutaneous nerve, has the largest share of the flexion force. It arises flat on the humeral shaft and inserts on the ulnar tuberosity. The radial nerve is located on its lateral edge and medial to the brachioradialis muscle.

References

1. Wegmann K, Burkhart KJ, Koslowsky TC, Koebke J, Neiss WF, Muller LP. Arterial supply of the distal humerus. Surg Radiol Anat. 2014;36(7):705–11. https://doi.org/10.1007/s00276-013-1240-z.
2. Kimball JP, Glowczewskie F, Wright TW. Intraosseous blood supply to the distal humerus. J Hand Surg Am. 2007;32(5):642–6. https://doi.org/10.1016/j.jhsa.2007.02.019.
3. Schub DL, Frisch NC, Bachmann KR, Winalski C, Saluan PM. Mapping of cartilage depth in the knee and elbow for use in osteochondral autograft procedures. Am J Sports Med. 2013;41(4):903–7. https://doi.org/10.1177/0363546513475343.
4. Morrey BF, Sanchez-Sotelo J. The elbow and its disorders. 4th ed. Philadelphia: Saunders; 2009.
5. Rahman RK, Levine WN, Ahmad CS. Elbow medial collateral ligament injuries. Curr Rev Musculoskelet Med. 2008;1(3–4):197–204. https://doi.org/10.1007/s12178-008-9026-3.
6. Buck FM, Zoner CS, Cardoso F, et al. Can osseous landmarks in the distal medial humerus be used to identify the attachment sites of ligaments and tendons: paleopathologic-anatomic imaging study in cadavers. Skeletal Radiol. 2010;39(9):905–13. https://doi.org/10.1007/s00256-009-0799-2.
7. Nagamoto H, Yamamoto N, Kurokawa D, et al. Evaluation of the thickness of the medial ulnar collateral ligament in junior high and high school baseball players. J Med Ultrason (2001). 2015;42(3):395–400. https://doi.org/10.1007/s10396-014-0605-1.
8. An KN, Morrey BF, Chao EY. The effect of partial removal of proximal ulna on elbow constraint. Clin Orthop Relat Res. 1986;(209):270–9.
9. Giannicola G, Sedati P, Cinotti G, Bullitta G, Polimanti D. The ulnar greater sigmoid notch "coverage angle": bone and cartilage contribution. Magnetic resonance imaging anatomic study on 78 elbows. J Shoulder Elbow Surg. 2015;24(12):1934–8. https://doi.org/10.1016/j.jse.2015.06.006.
10. Puchwein P, Schildhauer TA, Schoffmann S, Heidari N, Windisch G, Pichler W. Three-dimensional morphometry of the proximal ulna: a comparison to currently used anatomically preshaped ulna plates. J Shoulder Elb Surg. 2012;21(8):1018–23. https://doi.org/10.1016/j.jse.2011.07.004.
11. Ablove RH, Moy OJ, Howard C, Peimer CA, S'Doia S. Ulnar coronoid process anatomy: possible implications for elbow instability. Clin Orthop Relat Res. 2006;449:259–61. https://doi.org/10.1097/01.blo.0000218729.59838.bc.
12. Ramirez MA, Stein JA, Murthi AM. Varus posteromedial instability. Hand Clin. 2015;31(4):557–63. https://doi.org/10.1016/j.hcl.2015.06.005.
13. Hartzler RU, Llusa-Perez M, Steinmann SP, Morrey BF, Sanchez-Sotelo J. Transverse coronoid fracture: when does it have to be fixed? Clin Orthop Relat Res. 2014;472(7):2068–74. https://doi.org/10.1007/s11999-014-3477-1.
14. Terada N, Yamada H, Seki T, Urabe T, Takayama S. The importance of reducing small fractures of the coronoid process in the treatment of unstable elbow dislocation. J Shoulder Elb Surg. 2000;9(4):344–6. https://doi.org/10.1067/mse.2000.106082.
15. Irish SE, Langohr GD, Willing R, King GJ, Johnson JA. Implications of radial head hemiarthroplasty dish depth on radiocapitellar contact mechanics. J Hand Surg Am. 2015;40(4):723–9. https://doi.org/10.1016/j.jhsa.2015.01.030.
16. Alolabi B, Studer A, Gray A, et al. Selecting the diameter of a radial head implant: an assessment of local landmarks. J Shoulder Elb Surg. 2013;22(10):1395–9. https://doi.org/10.1016/j.jse.2013.04.005.
17. Patel BA. The hominoid proximal radius: re-interpreting locomotor behaviors in early hominins. J Hum Evol. 2005;48(4):415–32. https://doi.org/10.1016/j.jhevol.2005.01.001.
18. Green JB, Zelouf DS. Forearm instability. J Hand Surg Am. 2009;34(5):953–61. https://doi.org/10.1016/j.jhsa.2009.03.018.
19. Wegmann K, Müller LP. Knöcherne Verletzungen des Ellenbogens. Orthop Unfallchir up2date. 2012;7(5):339–64. https://doi.org/10.1055/s-0032-1324852.
20. Wegmann K, Dargel J, Burkhart KJ, Bruggemann GP, Muller LP. The Essex-Lopresti lesion. Strategies Trauma Limb Reconstr. 2012;7(3):131–9. https://doi.org/10.1007/s11751-012-0149-0.
21. Johnson JA, Beingessner DM, Gordon KD, Dunning CE, Stacpoole RA, King GJ. Kinematics and stability of the fractured and implant-reconstructed radial head. J Shoulder Elb Surg. 2005;14(1 Suppl S):195S–201S. https://doi.org/10.1016/j.jse.2004.09.034.
22. Lanting BA, Ferreira LM, Johnson JA, Athwal GS, King GJ. The effect of excision of the radial head and metallic radial head replacement on the tension in the interosseous membrane. Bone Joint J. 2013;95-B(10):1383–7. https://doi.org/10.1302/0301-620X.95B10.31844.
23. Sanal HT, Chen L, Haghighi P, Trudell DJ, Resnick DL. Annular ligament of the elbow: MR arthrography appearance with anatomic and histologic correlation. AJR Am J Roentgenol. 2009;193(2):W122–6. https://doi.org/10.2214/AJR.08.1887.
24. Wegmann K, Hain MK, Ries C, Neiss WF, Muller LP, Burkhart KJ. Do the radial head prosthesis components fit with the anatomical structures of the proximal radioulnar joint? Surg Radiol Anat. 2015;37(7):743–7. https://doi.org/10.1007/s00276-014-1407-2.
25. Moritomo H, Murase T, Arimitsu S, Oka K, Yoshikawa H, Sugamoto K. The in vivo isometric point of the lateral ligament of the elbow. J Bone Joint Surg Am. 2007;89(9):2011–7. https://doi.org/10.2106/JBJS.F.00868.
26. O'Brien MJ, Savoie FH 3rd. Arthroscopic and open management of posterolateral rotatory instability of the elbow. Sports Med Arthrosc Rev. 2014;22(3):194–200. https://doi.org/10.1097/JSA.0000000000000029.

27. O'Driscoll SW, Bell DF, Morrey BF. Posterolateral rotatory instability of the elbow. J Bone Joint Surg Am. 1991;73(3):440–6.
28. Wegmann K, Burkhart KJ, Bingoel AS, Ries C, Neiss WF, Muller LP. Anatomic relations between the lateral collateral ligament and the radial head: implications for arthroscopic resection of the synovial fold of the elbow. Knee Surg Sports Traumatol Arthrosc. 2015;23(11):3421–5. https://doi.org/10.1007/s00167-014-3091-5.
29. Haapaniemi T, Berggren M, Adolfsson L. Complete transection of the median and radial nerves during arthroscopic release of post-traumatic elbow contracture. Arthroscopy. 1999;15(7):784–7.
30. Leong NL, Cohen JR, Lord E, Wang JC, McAllister DR, Petrigliano FA. Demographic trends and complication rates in arthroscopic elbow surgery. Arthroscopy. 2015;31(10):1928–32. https://doi.org/10.1016/j.arthro.2015.03.036.
31. Nelson GN, Wu T, Galatz LM, Yamaguchi K, Keener JD. Elbow arthroscopy: early complications and associated risk factors. J Shoulder Elb Surg. 2014;23(2):273–8. https://doi.org/10.1016/j.jse.2013.09.026.
32. Hackl M, Lappen S, Burkhart KJ, et al. Elbow positioning and joint insufflation substantially influence median and radial nerve locations. Clin Orthop Relat Res. 2015;473(11):3627–34. https://doi.org/10.1007/s11999-015-4442-3.
33. Hackl M, Lappen S, Burkhart KJ, Neiss WF, Muller LP, Wegmann K. The course of the median and radial nerve across the elbow: an anatomic study. Arch Orthop Trauma Surg. 2015;135(7):979–83. https://doi.org/10.1007/s00402-015-2228-4.
34. Hackl M, Wegmann K, Lappen S, Helf C, Burkhart KJ, Muller LP. The course of the posterior interosseous nerve in relation to the proximal radius: is there a reliable landmark? Injury. 2015;46(4):687–92. https://doi.org/10.1016/j.injury.2015.01.028.
35. Contreras MG, Warner MA, Charboneau WJ, Cahill DR. Anatomy of the ulnar nerve at the elbow: potential relationship of acute ulnar neuropathy to gender differences. Clin Anat. 1998;11(6):372–8.
36. von Schroeder HP, Scheker LR. Redefining the "Arcade of Struthers". J Hand Surg Am. 2003;28(6):1018–21.
37. Karatas A, Apaydin N, Uz A, Tubbs R, Loukas M, Gezen F. Regional anatomic structures of the elbow that may potentially compress the ulnar nerve. J Shoulder Elb Surg. 2009;18(4):627–31. https://doi.org/10.1016/j.jse.2009.03.004.
38. Molinier F, Laffosse JM, Bouali O, Tricoire JL, Moscovici J. The anconeus, an active lateral ligament of the elbow: new anatomical arguments. Surg Radiol Anat. 2011;33(7):617–21. https://doi.org/10.1007/s00276-010-0767-5.
39. Pereira BP. Revisiting the anatomy and biomechanics of the anconeus muscle and its role in elbow stability. Ann Anat. 2013;195(4):365–70. https://doi.org/10.1016/j.aanat.2012.05.007.

Documentation of Elbow Arthroscopy

2

Alexander Ellwein, Helmut Lill,
and Andreas Lenich

Contents

A. Ellwein (✉) · H. Lill
DIAKOVERE Friederikenstift, Hannover, Germany
e-mail: alexander.ellwein@diakovere.de;
Helmut.Lill@diakovere.de

A. Lenich
Zentrum für Ellenbogen und Schulter Therapie im
Ortivity MVZ Orthopädie am Stiglmaierplatz,
München, Germany

A. B. Imhoff, A. Lenich (eds.), *Elbow Arthroscopy and Minimal Invasive Surgery*,
https://doi.org/10.1007/978-3-031-75611-5_2

2.1 Checklist (Fig. 2.1)

Diagnostic arthroscopy of the elbow

Diagnosis

____

1. Side

- o **Right**
- o **Left**

2. Anesthesia

- o **Regional anesthesia**
- o **General anesthesia**

3. Examination under anesthesia

Ext/Flex pre-OP ____/____/____

Pro/Sup pre-OP ____/____/____

0° medial	-	+	++	+++
30° medial	-	+	++	+++
0° lateral	-	+	++	+++
30° lateral	-	+	++	+++

Ext/Flex post-OP ____/____/____

Pro/Sup post-OP ____/____/____

4. Positioning

- o Supine
- o Lateral
- o Prone

5. Tourniquet

- o Tourniquet (__mmHg)
- o No

6. Preparation

- o Landmarks
- o Insuflation of the joint
- o Insertion of canula

7. Image documentation

7.1. View from high dorsoradial portal

- o Tip of the olecranon
- o Olecaranon fossa
- o Medial recess
- o Lateral recess

7.2. View from high dorsoradial through the dorsolateral recess

- o Humeroradial plica
- o Humeroradial articulation
- o Humeroulnar articulation
- o Radioulnar articulation

7.3. View from anteromedial/anterolateral

- o Radius head
- o Capitulum
- o Coronoid process
- o Annular ligament

8. Cartilage quality (Outerbridge)

- o CM 0°: Normal finding
- o CM I°: Softening of the cartilage surface
- o CM II°: small cuts
- o CM III°: Lesion involves >50 % of the thickness
- o CM IV°: exposed subchondral bone

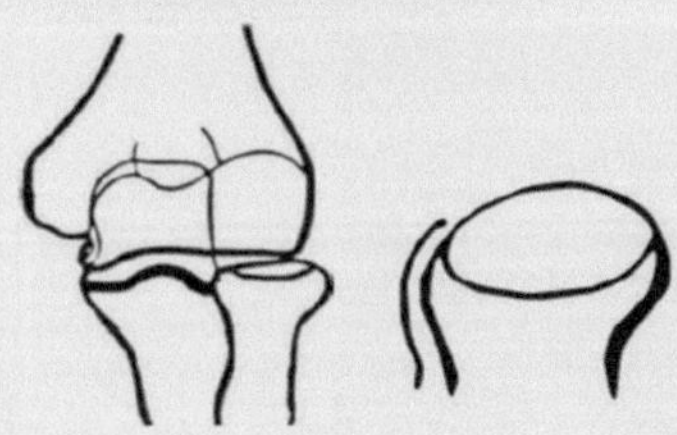

Fig. 2.1 Diagnostic tour checklist. Abbreviation: *Ext* extension, *Flex* flexion, *Pro* pronation, *Sup* supination, *CM* chondromalacia, *MCL* medial collateral ligament, *LCL* lateral collateral ligament, *PLRI* posterolateral rotatory instability

9. Plica radiohumeral

- Radius head not covered
- Radius head about 1/3 covered
- Radius head about 2/3 covered
- Radius head completely covered bedeckt

10. Synovialitis

- No
- Local
- Generalized
- Extensive

11. 11. Osteophytic additions to the tip of the olecranon (removal of the tip of the olecranon from the cartilage-bone border at the 90 ° flexed elbow)

- ≤6 mm
- >6 mm

12. Free joint loose bodies

- No
- Dorsal compartment
- Medial Recess
- Lateral Recess
- Ventral compartment

13. 3. Instability diagnostics (with 4-mm rod)

13.1. Humeroulnar dorsal

13.1.1. Medial third (MCL)

- 0 mm (resilient resistance)
- 2 mm (penetration of the tip)
- 4 mm (complete penetration)

13.1.2. Lateral third (LCL)

- 0–4 mm (up to 1 switching stick)
- 4–8 mm (up to 2 switching stick)
- >8 mm (>2 switching stick)

13.1.3. Central third (LCL + MCL)

- 0 mm (resilient resistance)
- 2 mm (penetration of the tip)
- 4 mm (complete penetration)

13.2. Humeroulnar ventral (PLRI)

- 0–4 mm (up to 1 switching stick)
- 4–6 mm (up to 1,5 switching stick)
- 6–8 mm (up to 2 switching stick)
- >8 mm (subluxation, coronoid is visible)

13.3. Humeroradial

- 0 mm (resilient resistance)
- 2 mm (penetration of the tip)
- 4 mm (complete penetration)

13.4. Radioulnar (Lig. anulare)

- 0 mm (resilient resistance)
- 2 mm (penetration of the tip)
- 4 mm (complete penetration)

13.5. Joint incongruence trochlea and coronoid

- Joint congruent
- Radially opening
- Ulnar opening

13.6. Translation radius head to capitulum (PLRI)

- Centrally under the capitulum
- Dorsal shift: 1/4 joint surface
- Dorsal shift: 2/4 joint surface
- Dorsal shift: 3/4 joint surface
- Dorsal shift: 4/4 joint surface

Fig. 2.1 (continued)

2.2 Diagnoses of the Instability

Table 2.1 Ligaments evaluated during arthroscopic instability diagnostic

Joint	Injured band structure
Humeroradial grade 1	LUCL (lateral ulnar collateral ligament)
Humeroulnar grade 2	LUCL+ MCL (medial collateral ligament)
Humeroradial	LCL (lateral collateral ligament)
Radioulnar	Annular ligament

The structures to be tested for instability diagnostics are listed in Table 2.1:

3 Patient Positioning and Arthroscopic Portals

Lucca Lacheta and Sebastian Siebenlist

Contents

3.1 Anesthesia

General anesthesia is more comfortable for both the patient and the surgeon than plexus or regional anesthesia. With general anesthesia, optimal relaxation can be achieved and it allows the immediate postoperative examination of the neurological status. Depending on the surgical indication (e.g., in arthrolysis), general anesthesia can be combined with regional anesthesia (interscalene or infraclavicular block).

3.1.1 Positioning

Before positioning of the patient takes place, the surgeon should always perform an examination of the elbow joint under anesthesia and compare the diseased side with the contralateral side [1]. The range of motion as well as the stability of the joint should be assessed and compared with previous findings when the patient was awake. The surgeon should position the patient by himself to ensure the possibility of accessing all the articular compartments. In addition, the joint must be

L. Lacheta · S. Siebenlist (✉)
Department of Orthopaedic Sports Medicine, Klinikum Rechts der Isar, Technical University of Munich, Munich, Germany
e-mail: Lucca.Lacheta@charite.de; Sebastian.Siebenlist@tum.de

A. B. Imhoff, A. Lenich (eds.), *Elbow Arthroscopy and Minimal Invasive Surgery*, https://doi.org/10.1007/978-3-031-75611-5_3

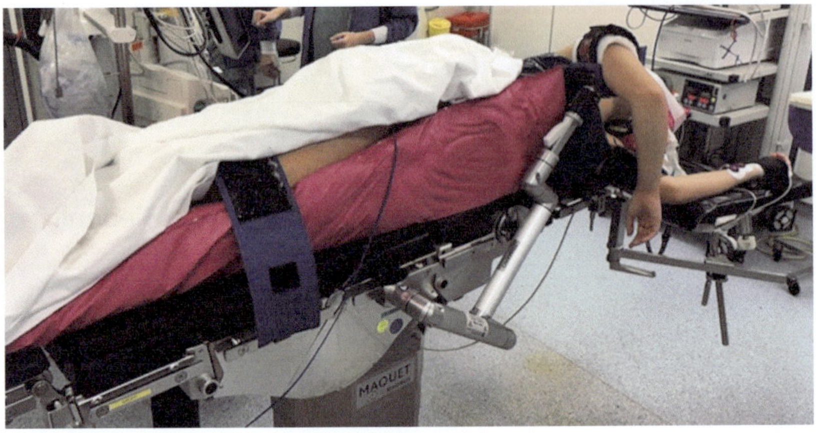

Fig. 3.1 Lateral positioning supported by the vacuum mattress

freely movable in extension and flexion as well as in pronation and supination. The patient can be positioned in a prone, supine, or lateral decubitus position.

3.1.1.1 Lateral Positioning

The authors prefer the lateral position; the patient lies on his healthy side in a vacuum mattress (Fig. 3.1). The pelvis and the thorax are secured by the vacuum mattress, and soft gel mats are placed between the legs. Good padding of the shoulder and head and aligned positioning of the cervical spine must be strictly respected. The operated arm should be stabilized in a hydraulic arm holder. The 90-degree flexed elbow joint must be freely accessible on all sides and mobile in a full range of motion (Fig. 3.2). According to the surgeon's preference, a tourniquet padded with cotton is applied to the upper arm. The lateral position allows optimal working conditions for the ventral and dorsal joint compartments. For the arthroscopic beginners, the reversed anatomy is disadvantageous and requires habituation. By adding a sterile side table, arthroscopic operation can be converted easily to an open procedure (Fig. 3.3). In the lateral position, the procedure may take more time, but offers a good option for switching to an open procedure.

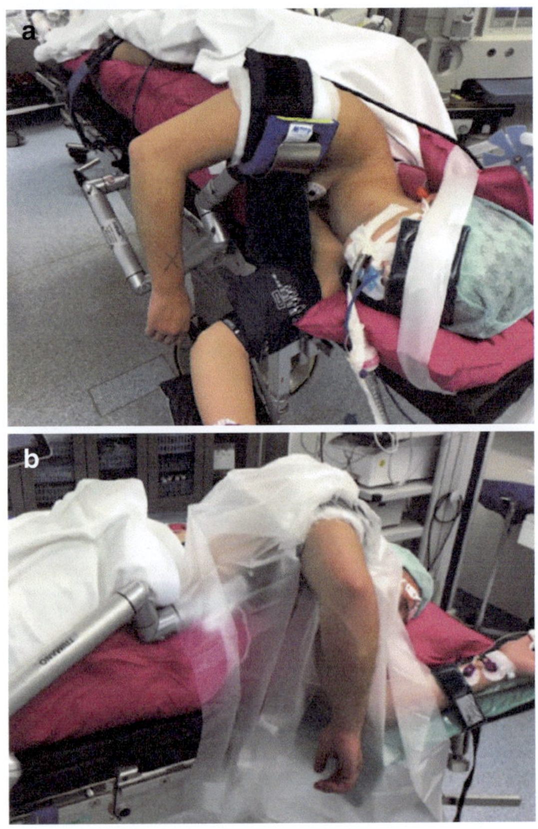

Fig. 3.2 (**a**) The operated arm is positioned in a hydraulic arm holder. (**b**) Before disinfecting, the arm is covered with a foil to prevent the disinfectant from flowing under the tourniquet

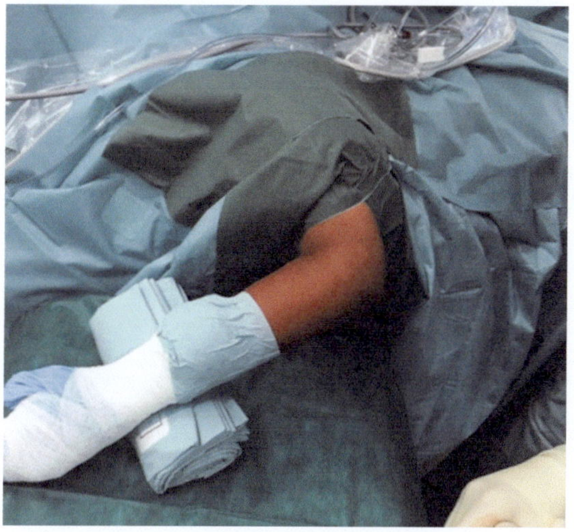

Fig. 3.3 Lateral positioning: the arm to be operated is repositioned on a sterile side table for an open lateral approach

3.1.1.2 Prone Position

The prone position offers the surgeon the same advantages in terms of access and work opportunities as the lateral position. The upper arm of the patient is abducted to 90 degrees, the shoulder joint is attached to arm support on one side of the operating table. Good padding of the arm is recommended.

It is also advisable to secure the upper arm on the arm support, for example, with a plaster or tape to avoid slipping of the arm. Changing the position of the anesthetized patient in the prone position, the uncomfortable lying of the patient, and the difficult anesthesia conditions in case of a conversion to general anesthesiea are disadvantageous for regional anesthesia in comparison with the lateral position. Padding of the chest and pelvis is mandatory for adequate ventilation.

3.2 Arthroscopy Portals

It is recommended to mark the main anatomical landmarks, endangered structures, and portals before every elbow arthroscopy after positioning, disinfection, and draping of the arm to be treated. The standard portals and relevant anatomical structures are summarized in Table 3.1. The monitor or arthroscopy tower is placed opposite to the elbow to be operated (Fig. 3.4). A 4.0-mm lens is used as standard, and the pump pressure is adjusted to 40 mmHg. The surgeon should control the presence of all the arthroscopic instruments before starting the arthroscopy (see overview).

Instrument Set

- Instrument
- Marker pen
- Puncture cannula
- 20 mL syringe
- Mosquito clamp
- Scissors
- Grasping forceps/rongeur
- Probe
- Switching stick, if necessary interchangeable trocar
- Retractors
- Shaver
- Diathermy
- Inflow cannula
- Working cannula
- Microfracture awls
- Curettes
- Chisel/osteotome
- Optional: 2.7 mm optic for small joints

The joint should be filled with fluid before incising the first portal to distend the joint capsule and push the neurovascular structures as far as possible from the joint [2]. The joint filling can be done through soft spot or transtriceps portals (Fig. 3.5). If the cannula is correctly placed intraarticularly, with a proper filling of the capsule with fluid, a U-shaped protrusion around the olecranon is visible and the elbow will extend approximately 10–20°. After the cannula is removed, a jet flow of the fluid can confirm that the filling occurred in the intraarticular space.

3.2.1 Anterolateral Portal

The anterolateral portal is 1–2 cm ventral and 2 cm proximal to the lateral humeral epicondyle, between the radius head and the ventral part of

Table 3.1 Arthroscopy portals

Portal	Location	Endangered structures	Tips and tricks
Anterolateral	2 cm ventral and proximal to the lateral humeral epicondyle	Radial nerve, posterior antebrachial cutaneous nerve	Only skin incision with scalpel, blunt preparation over the capsule, sharp perforation of the capsule
Anteromedial	2 cm ventral and proximal to the medial humeral epicondyle	Median nerve, medial antebrachial continuous nerve	Inside-out shuttle maneuver
Posterior central	2–3 cm central and proximal to the tip of that olecranon, trans-tendon	Ulnar nerve, posterior antiebrachial cutaneous nerve	With a scalpel through all tissues in the fossa, if needed ulnar shifting for better accessibility of the ulnar recess
High posterolateral	1–2 cm proximal to the tip of the olecranon, lateral edge of that triceps tendon	Posterior antebrachial cutaneous nerve	With a scalpel through all layers of tissue—Introducing the trocar via switching stick
Deep posterior [soft spot]	Triangle formed by the radius, tip of the olecranon, and lateral humeral epicondyle	Posterior antebrachial cutaneous nerve	If needed, the camera portal for a better view of radiocapitellar and ulnohumeral

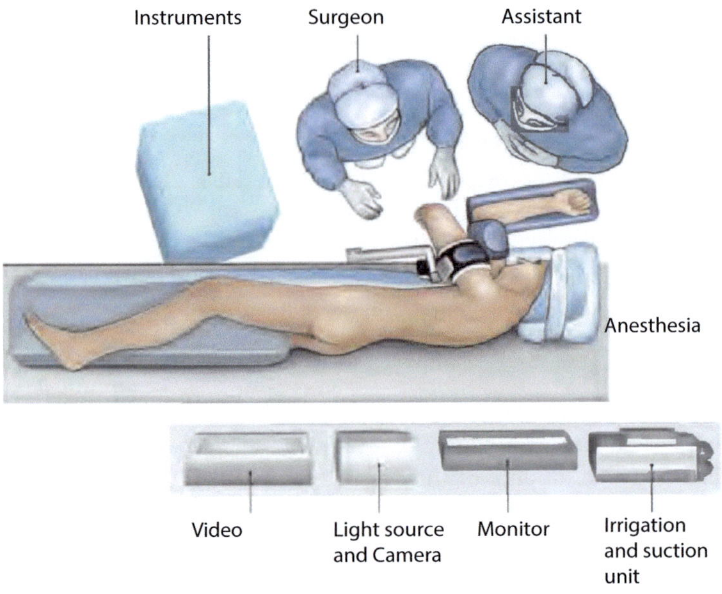

Fig. 3.4 Set-up of the elbow arthroscopy

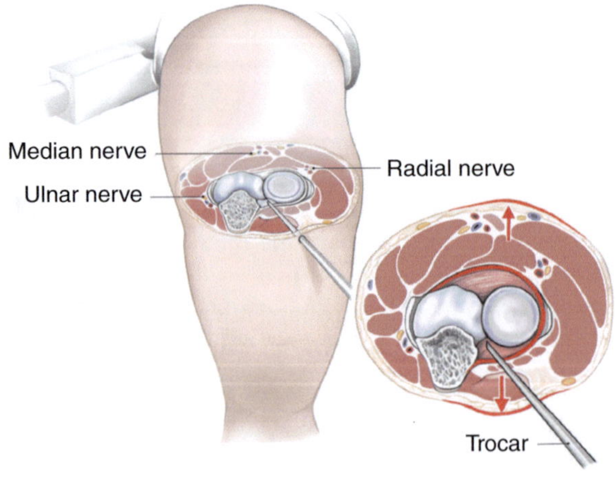

Fig. 3.5 Filling up the joint in front of the first portal system using the "soft-spot portal"

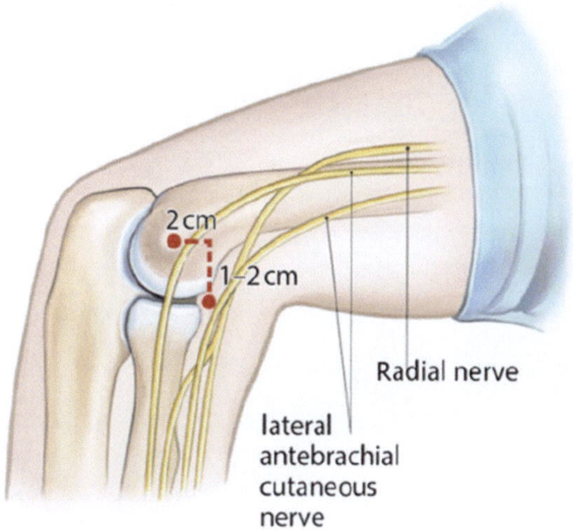

Fig. 3.6 Anterolateral portal

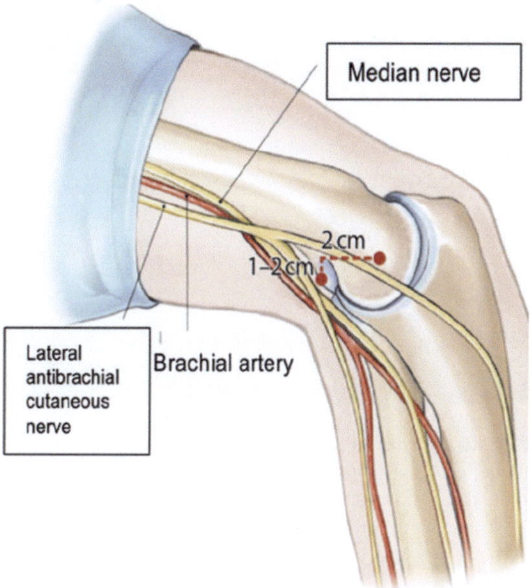

Fig. 3.7 Anteromedial portal

the capitulum (Fig. 3.6). To protect the surrounding neurovascular structures, it is recommended to just incise the skin with a scalpel and then dissect bluntly (e.g., with a clamp or scissors) on the joint capsule. Then, the capsule perforated with the trocar (aiming at the coronoid process), and a loss of resistance is usually felt after penetration of the capsule with the trocar.

The anterolateral portal enables you to view the coronoid process, the coronoid fossa, the trochlea, the medial part of the capsule, as well as the radius head and the ventral part of the proximal radioulnar joint. A deviation of the portal must be avoided due to the proximity of the radial nerve and posterior cutaneous antebrachial nerve. When placing the portal more distally, the distance to the radial nerve is significantly reduced [3]. The anterolateral portal is used as the primary portal for inserting an inflow cannula; with the correct placement of the cannula, the previously injected fluid in the soft spot will flow accordingly.

3.2.2 Anteromedial Portal

This standard portal is about 1–2 cm ventral and 2 cm proximal to the medial humeral epicondyle and is used as both viewing and working portal (Fig. 3.7). The location of this portal can vary according to the indication of the operation. The location of the medial antebrachial cutaneous nerve and the median nerve should be taken into consideration. Directly anterior to the location of this portal lies the course of the ulnar nerve, the ulnar nerve can be palpated very closely. For possible anterior subluxation of the ulnar nerve or in the case of anterior transposition of the ulnar nerve, the nerve must be exposed and kept away from the portal. When working in the anterior compartment of the joint, the cannula can be a helpful guide to the surgeon.

Via the anteromedial portal, the radial head, the capitulum, the trochlea, the coronoid process, the anterolateral capsule portions, and the annular ligament can be assessed.

For the anteromedial portal two techniques are used:

1. Outside-in-technique:

   The camera is used to show the anteromedial capsule. From the outside, probing with the use of a cannula directed toward the center of the elbow is performed. A skin incision is done over it, and then blunt preparation and trocar insertion are done to promote the appli-

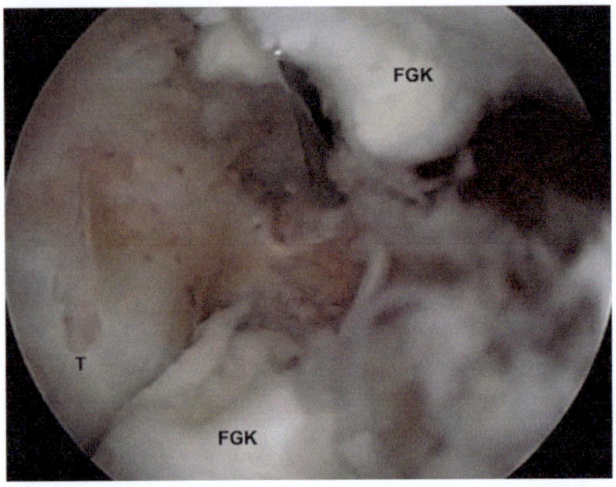

Fig. 3.8 Anteromedial portal placement in outside-in technique: probing the portal position with a cannula to determine the working angle. *FGK* free loose body, *T* trochlea

cation of the anterolateral portal. The advantage of this technique is the good assessment of the portal positions and the exact determination of the instrument's working angle (Fig. 3.8).

2. Inside-out technique:

   The optic is inserted all the way to the anteromedial joint capsule. Then, the optic is replaced by a switching stick, the medial joint capsule is pierced, and the switching stick is advanced medially through the subcutaneous tissue (Fig. 3.9). With the aid of the switching stick, the optic trocar can be inserted over it.

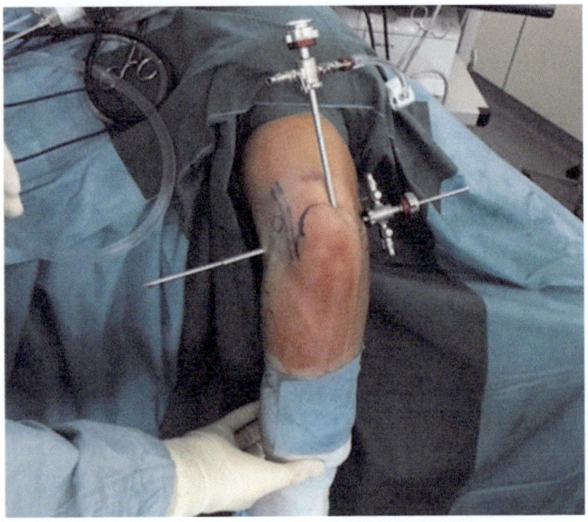

Fig. 3.9 Anteromedial portal placement using the inside-out technique: the trocar is "shuttled" from lateral to medial with the aid of the switching stick. The inflow for joint distension is continuously maintained during the shuttle maneuver via the second trocar with connected water tube (high posterolateral portal)

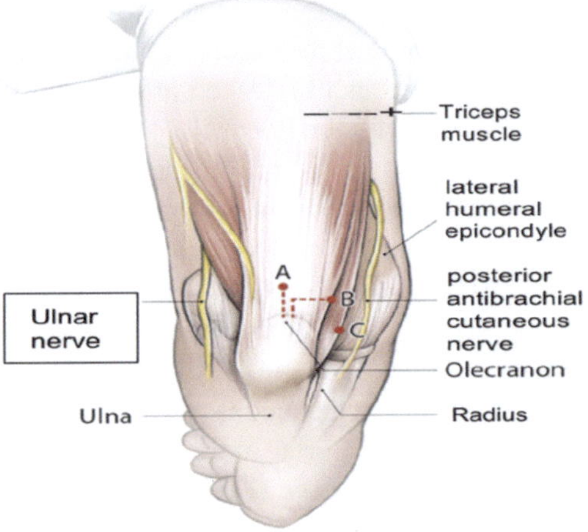

Fig. 3.10 Posterior portal: posterocentral portal (A), high posterolateral portal (B), and deep posterolateral portal (soft spot; C)

3.2.3 Posterocentral Portal

The posterocentral portal (synonym: superoposterior or transtricipital portal) is approximately 3–4 cm proximal to the olecranon tip, central through the tendon of the triceps brachii muscle (Fig. 3.10). After probing toward the olecranon fossa, an incision is done with a scalpel under arthroscopic control, directed to the fossa.

The transtricipital portal serves as the primary working portal for the dorsal joint space. Particularly, for the removal of posteromedial osteophytes of the olecranon, it is often required to place the portal a little bit medially to fully reach the ulnar recess. In these cases, the ulnar nerve should be kept away through a mini-incision to be able to work safely (Fig. 3.11).

In special cases, the posterocentral portal can also be used as a viewing portal to the dorsal joint parts such as olecranon, olecranon fossa, and ulnar recess.

3.2.4 High Posterolateral Portal

It is located approximately 1–2 cm proximal to the olecranon tip immediately on the lateral edge of the triceps tendon. With a scalpel, an incision is made through all tissue layers, along the fiber's direction, directly toward the olecranon fossa (Fig. 3.10). The switching stick is inserted till bone contact is felt.

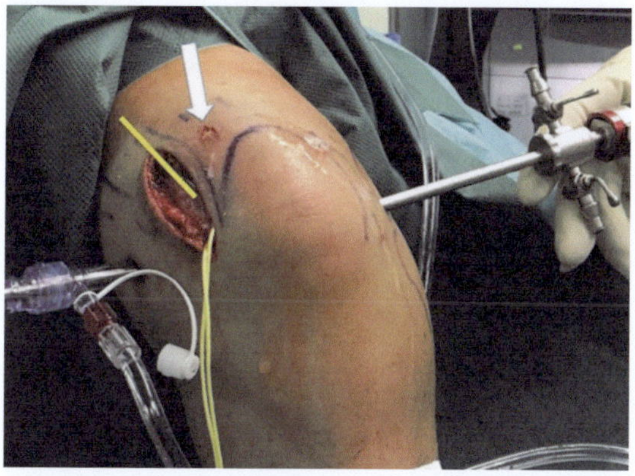

Fig. 3.11 Very close relationship of the ulnar nerve (yellow bar) to the medially displaced transtricipital portal (white arrow)

Possible adhesions can be bluntly removed, thereby increasing the capsule volume. Then, the trocar is placed over the switching stick. When perforating the joint capsule, loss of resistance is felt and not infrequently a "snap" is heard. Furthermore, the leakage of fluid can be observed with an already connected rinsing fluid system. Insertion of the optic is done, after being sure that the trocar is intraarticular. Through the high posterolateral portal, the olecranon tip, the olecranon fossa, and the collateral recesses can be assessed (Fig. 3.11). When advancing the optic over the lateral recess along the lateral olecranon edge, the dorsal capitulum, the dorsal radius head, and the humeroulnar joint can be visible (Fig. 3.12).

3.2.5 Deep Posterolateral Portal ("Soft Spot")

The deep posterolateral portal corresponds to the dorsoradial soft spot and is in the center between the radius head, olecranon, and lateral epicondyle (Fig. 3.10). The posterior antebrachial cutaneous nerve is in close proximity to this portal. To place

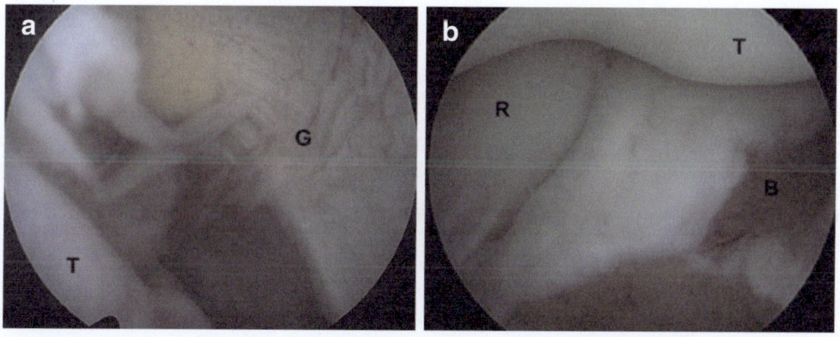

Fig. 3.12 (**a**) Ulnar recess: posteromedial joint capsule (G), dorsal trochlea (T). (**b**) View in the so-called triangle between the humeroulnar joint "bare area" (B)—cartilage-free zone of the olecranon, trochlea humeri (T), and radial head (R) via the high posterolateral portal

this portal, the camera is set distally under vision through the posterolateral portal, and a puncture with a cannula in the desired portal position is done. Then, the skin is incised, and blunt dissection with scissors is done.

The soft-spot portal is primarily used as a working portal (e.g., shaver) for the posterolateral area, but it can be also used as a viewing portal to improve the viewing angle in the radiocapitalellar joint or humeroulnar joint (Fig. 3.13), especially in the case of osteochondral lesions in the capitulum or arthroscopic treatment of radial head fractures.

3.2.6 Accessory Portals

Additional portals are used for certain indications (e.g., arthroscopic arthrolysis). The proximal anterolateral portal is approximately 1–2 cm more proximal to the "classic" anterolateral portal and aims at the center of the elbow [4] (Fig. 3.14). The proximal anteromedial portal (synonym: superomedial portal) is approximately 1 cm proximal to the anteromedial standard portal [5]. Compared to other portals, this portal is safer; so, in the literature, it is recommended to use it as an initial portal (especially with little experience in prone or lateral position; [6]).

Systematic Approach

Systematic, diagnostic arthroscopy of the elbow (Figs. 3.15, 3.16, and 3.17).

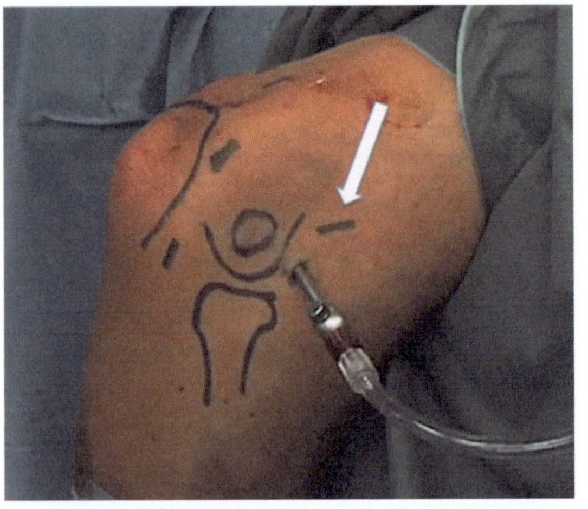

Fig. 3.14 The inflow canula is located in the anterolateral standard portal. The arrow points to the additional proximal anterolateral portal

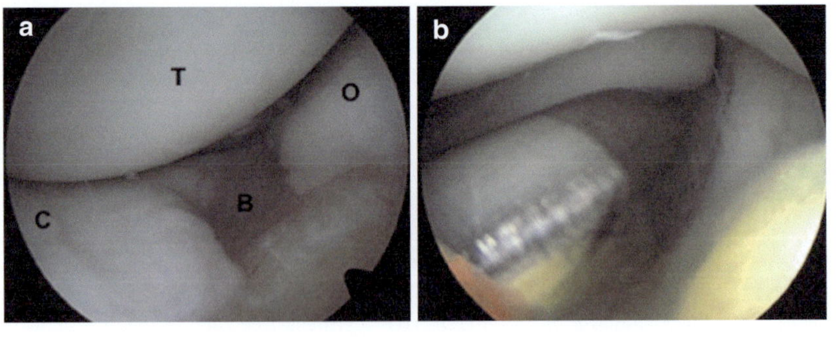

Fig. 3.13 (**a**) View of the humeroular joint through the deep posterolateral portal. *O* olecranon, *T* trochlea, *B* "bare area." (**b**) Stability test using the scaled switching stick via the soft-spot portal (view through the high posterolateral portal)

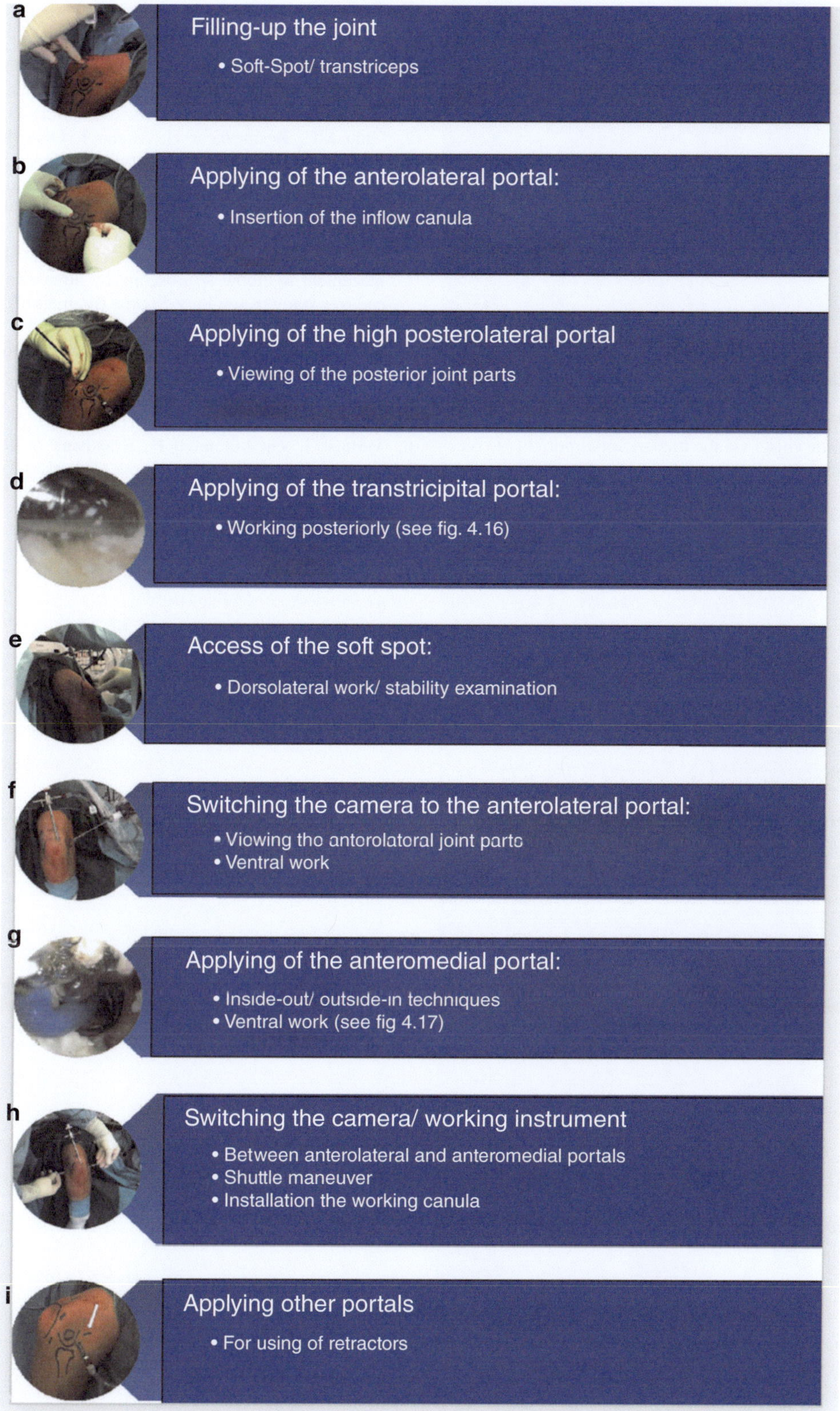
a
Filling-up the joint
• Soft-Spot/ transtriceps
b
Applying of the anterolateral portal:
• Insertion of the inflow canula
c
Applying of the high posterolateral portal
• Viewing of the posterior joint parts
d
Applying of the transtricipital portal:
• Working posteriorly (see fig. 4.16)
e
Access of the soft spot:
• Dorsolateral work/ stability examination
f
Switching the camera to the anterolateral portal:
• Viowing tho antorolatoral joint partc
• Ventral work
g
Applying of the anteromedial portal:
• Inside-out/ outside-in techniques
• Ventral work (see fig 4.17)
h
Switching the camera/ working instrument
• Between anterolateral and anteromedial portals
• Shuttle maneuver
• Installation the working canula
i
Applying other portals
• For using of retractors

Fig. 3.15 (a–i) Flowchart: systematic diagnostic tour

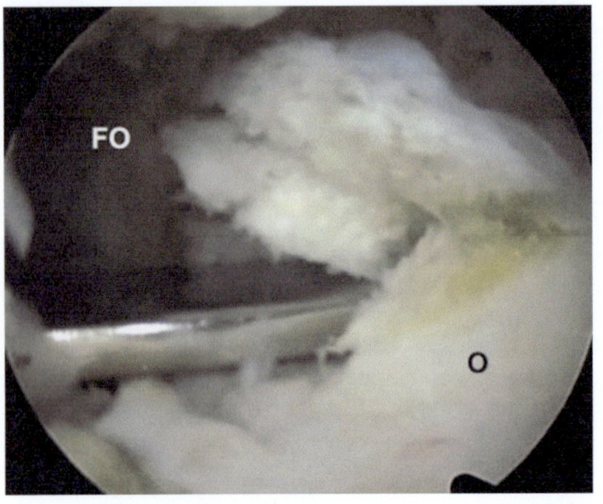

Fig. 3.16 Osteophyte removal at the tip of the olecranon (O) with the chisel via the transtricipital portal (*FO* olecranon fossa)

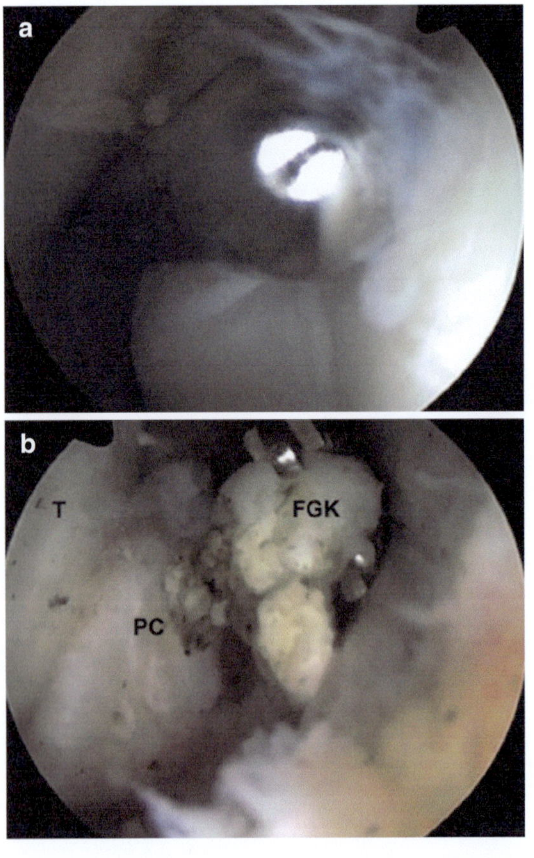

Fig. 3.17 (**a**, **b**) Removal of capsular adhesions with the soft tissue shaver. *T* trochlea, *FGK* free loose body

References

1. O'Driscoll SW, Lawton RL, Smith AM. The "moving valgus stress test" for medial collateral ligament tears of the elbow. Am J Sports Med. 2005;33(2):231–9.
2. Unlu MC, Kesmezacar H, Akgun I, Ogut T, Uzun I. Anatomic relationship between elbow arthroscopy portals and neurovascular structures in different elbow and forearm positions. J Shoulder Elb Surg. 2006;15(4):457–62.
3. Claessen FM, Kachooei AR, Kolovich GP, et al. Portal placement in elbow arthroscopy by novice surgeons: cadaver study. Knee Surg Sports Traumatol Arthrosc. 2017;25(7):2247–54.
4. Noonburg GE, Baker CL Jr. Elbow arthroscopy. Instr Course Lect. 2006;55:87–93.
5. Lindenfeld TN. Medial approach in elbow arthroscopy. Am J Sports Med. 1990;18(4):413–7.
6. Verhaar J, van Mameren H, Brandsma A. Risks of neurovascular injury in elbow arthroscopy: starting anteromedially or anterolaterally? Arthroscopy. 1991;7(3):287–90.

Concepts of Arthroscopic Treatment of Osteochondral Lesions of the Elbow

4

S. Vogt and F. Blanke

Contents

S. Vogt (✉)
Department of Orthopaedic Sports Medicine Hessing Foundation, Augsburg, Germany
e-mail: Stephan.vogt@hessing-stiftung.de

F. Blanke
Department of Knee-, Shoulder-, Hip- and Elbow-Surgery, Schön Clinic München-Harlaching, München, Germany
e-mail: fblanke@schoen-klinik.de

4.1 Background

An osteochondral lesion (OCL) of the elbow joint is rare if compared to other joints and most frequently located at the capitulum humeri [1, 2]. It mainly affects young people performing activities like throwing and overhead sports.

The OCL of the elbow is mainly described in the literature among young baseball players, and therefore it is published in the American and Japanese literature [3–6]. Since the underlying genesis of this disease are usually microtraumata, it is appropriate to classify it as an osteochondral lesion and not as an osteochondrosis dissecans (OD).

A. B. Imhoff, A. Lenich (eds.), *Elbow Arthroscopy and Minimal Invasive Surgery*,
https://doi.org/10.1007/978-3-031-75611-5_4

To distinguish the OCL from Panner's disease, it has to be underlined that Panner's disease is a juvenile osteonecrosis of the entire capitulum [7]. Its equivalent in the hip joint is Perthes' disease [8]. It mainly occurs in boys under 10 years old and has a benign course [9]. Conservative therapy is the treatment of choice.

4.2 Etiology

Franz König, a German surgeon (1832–1910), was the first to describe the osteochondrosis dissecans in 1888 (OD; [10]). He assumed that the cause of this disease was a subchondral inflammatory process with the formation of a free chondral body. The exact aetiopathogenesis of the OD has not been clarified [1, 11]. Besides the inflammatory process, (micro)-traumatic and vascular reasons as well as genetic factors were discussed [12–15]. Because of several existing pathological mechanisms and multifactorial causes, the OD is not a clearly defined disease. That is the reason why this disease in the elbow joint should be referred to as an osteochondral lesion (OCL). It is assumed that repetitive traumata in the capitulum lead to an osteochondral lesion [9, 14–16].

The main causes are shear and compressive forces on the humeroradial joint which occur during the acceleration and deceleration phases in throwing sports [16]. Due to the high repetitive stresses in the elbow of throwing athletes, fatigue of the medial stabilizing muscles will occur, and this will result in an additional nonphysiological force on the secondary valgus and radiocapitular stabilizers of the elbow [1].

This hypothesis is supported by the increased incidence of this disease in the dominant limb of the throwing athletes. Schenk and co-authors found a significantly higher stiffness in the central part of the capitulum in relation to the lateral part in a cadaveric study. This mismatch between the different joint parts might be responsible for the formation of an osteochondral lesion of the capitulum [14].

4.3 Clinical Presentation

Patients often complain about load-dependent lateral elbow pain and a restriction of movements. The dominant extremity is mostly affected, and the pain increases with stress and loading of the joint and will usually improve after rest [15, 17]. An osteochondral lesion mainly affects adolescents and both genders. However, in countries like Japan and the United States, boys are more affected because a particularly large number of boys play baseball. Mechanical symptoms with a recurrent locking phenomenon (fragment dislocation) are frequently observed and are common in advanced grades of this disease [9].

4.4 Examination

In the clinical examination, tenderness over the capitulum, crepitation, and lateral joint pain under forced supination and pronation with axial compression are observed [9, 15]. Occasionally, an extension deficit and a slight joint effusion exist [12, 17, 18].

In addition to the evaluation of the range of motion, an examination of the medial and posterolateral stability of the elbow should always be performed [1].

4.5 Imaging and Classification

X-rays in anteroposterior (a.p.) and lateral (lat.) views as well as in a.p. view in 45° flexion should be performed to provide a better view into the humeroradial joint [1, 19].

In the early stages of the disease, the X-ray diagnostics are usually unremarkable. In advanced stages, irregularity of the capitulum with the appearance of sclerotic zones around the OCL can be observed. In case of fragment dislocation or separation, a loose body and bone defect can be recognized [1]. An MRI scan should be added to the X-ray diagnostics for a better assessment of the extent, stability, and vitality of the OCL fragment.

For MR imaging, the application of an intravenous contrast medium is recommended. In contrast to X-ray diagnostics, the MRI allows the diagnosis of the early stages of the disease and provides an exact classification of the lesion according to Nelson and Dipaola [20, 21]. This classification system was initially used to classify the osteochondral lesions of the knee and of the talus; however, in the meantime, it is increasingly used for the classification of osteochondral lesions of the elbow [2, 6, 17, 21]. Takahara et al. [19] suggested a simplified and more practical classification system for osteochondral lesions of the elbow. They divided the lesions into stable and unstable lesions. The stable lesions are those that usually heal spontaneously without surgery, and they are characterized by open growth plates, flattening of the capitulum, increased X-ray permeability, and free joint mobility. By contrast, unstable lesions are defined by closed growth plates, fragmentation of the lesion, and restriction of movement of more than 20°. In unstable lesions, the operative treatment has significantly better results.

4.6 Therapy

The decision between a surgical or nonsurgical treatment depends on the stability of the OCL and the width of the growth plates. Stable osteochondral lesions (no loose fragments and open growth plates) are usually treated conservatively, whereas unstable lesions (loose fragments and closed growth plates) should be treated surgically [3, 4, 12, 15, 19]. Contrary to the osteochondral lesions of the knee joint, the epiphyseal plate status in the elbow does not consistently affect the healing potential of the lesions. Some authors reported better results after conservative therapy in patients with open epiphyseal plates [3, 19], while other authors did not see such a correlation [18, 22]. Despite the contradictory data, in our opinion, the status of the epiphyseal plates is an important predictor for the healing potential of an osteochondral lesion, and the evaluation of the width of the growth plates significantly affects our treatment concept.

4.6.1 Conservative Therapy

Conservative therapy primarily includes a load modification with strict avoidance of pain-provoking activities and physiotherapeutic exercises to enhance the range of motion. We recommend returning to sport only in cases of complete healing of the OCL in the MRI.

Earlier studies of long-term results of the conservative therapy of the osteochondral lesions of the elbow showed residual complaints in more than half of all patients with secondary fragment dislocation and joint degeneration [22, 23]. However, in both study groups, no MRI imaging was performed for the diagnosis and classification of the osteochondral lesions.

By contrast, a recent publication by Mihara et al. supports conservative therapy for low-grade lesions [3]. The authors studied 39 baseball players with an average age of 12.8 years (follow-up period: 14.4 months). Complete healing was found in 25 of 30 patients with minor lesions, but only in 1 of 9 patients with high-grade lesions.

The results of the study of Takahara et al. showed that a successful conservative treatment is only possible with strict immobilization of the elbow and with the presence of open growth plates [19]. Patients with open growth plates who were treated with this regimen showed a complete healing of the lesion in 7 of 10 cases whereas patients with closed growth plates showed a complete healing only in 1 of 11 cases.

On the contrary, patients who continued full load bearing of the elbow showed inferior results regarding pain, X-ray morphology, and tissue regeneration even with open growth plates.

4.6.2 Surgical Treatment

The different options for surgical treatment are numerous and include arthroscopic debridement, microfracture or retrograde drilling, refixation of the fragment, an osteochondral transfer, or a matrix-induced chondrocyte transplantation (MACT) with cancellous bone plasty and osteotomies [2, 6, 12, 17–19, 24–27].

4.6.3 Arthroscopic Techniques

Several studies have been published in the last years and reported short- and medium-term results after arthroscopic fragment resection and defect debridement. They mostly showed good results regarding pain reduction, return to sports rate, and improvement of elbow mobility [6, 18, 25, 26].

By using the standard portals for elbow arthroscopy, the osteochondral lesion is evaluated. If the fragment is unstable (which is evaluated by probing the lesion), it should be removed. Subsequently, the defect area should be debrided using a shaver and a curette. Especially in young patients, this technique can be sufficient to produce bleeding and a secondary defect filling. Alternatively, a subtle subchondral bone opening (microfracture) can be performed. By using an awl with different curved angles, microholes are created in the defect, so that a bony bleeding is enhanced. Brownlow et al. evaluated 29 patients who received this surgical technique with an average follow-up of 77 months. Furthermore, 12 patients were pain-free, 14 patients complained of slight residual pain, and 3 patients complained of moderate pain. In addition, 81% of the patients could return to their previous level of sport after the surgery. However, 38% of the patients showed radiological signs of arthritis or loose bodies [24].

In other studies, arthroscopic refixation of the osteochondral fragment showed good results regarding fragment integration, pain, joint mobility, and return to sport rate [5, 15, 19]. However, this surgical technique is dependent on fragment and subchondral bone quality. Performing this technique, the fragment is first reduced and temporarily transfixed (e.g., with a K-wire). After that, the definitive refixation with cannulated screws (e.g., Leibinger system) is performed. The screws must be placed deep into the cartilage and should not have any contact with the opposite cartilage. Using this technique, Takahara et al. reported good results in 12 patients with a significant decrease in pain after fragment fixation [19].

4.6.4 Open Technique

As arthroscopic fragment resection, this procedure can also be performed by incision. This technique is technically not demanding and in contrast to arthroscopic resection, several long-term studies exist in the literature.

However, a high incidence of osteoarthritis and persistent complaints after surgery are evident, and revision surgery is frequently needed [19, 28].

Bauer et al. observed residual symptoms in 50% of the patients 23 years after open fragment resection and debridement. In 60% of the patients, a development of osteoarthritis was seen [28].

Osteochondral transfer has been increasingly performed in the last years in the treatment of osteochondral lesions of the elbow [2, 6, 17, 27]. The principle of this therapy is to replace the destroyed cartilage–bone complex with an autologous osteochondral cylinder, which is harvested from a "non-weight-bearing" area of the knee joint. The advantage of this technique is the complete autologous reconstruction of the articular surface of the joint with healthy hyaline cartilage and an intact subchondral bone.

The exposure of the capitulum is usually done via a lateral approach. The fascia between the anconeus muscle and the extensor carpi ulnaris muscle is incised. The joint capsule is exposed and opened at the level of the head of the radius. The annular ligament must be preserved. After visualizing the defect, its size is measured with a special instrument (e.g., OATS system, Arthrex, Naples, Florida). The recipient OATS chisel is advanced to the necessary depth (determined on the MRI). The removal of the cylinder is performed by rapid rotational movements (Fig. 4.1). The removed cylinder should be assessed as healthy throughout the whole circumference, to avoid the occurrence of osteonecrosis. If some sclerotic areas remain, these areas can be opened by drilling with a K-wire. Using a parapatellar lateral mini-arthrotomy, the proximal lateral trochlea is exposed and the donor cylinder is harvested. Then, the donor cylinder is inserted in the site of the lesion by press-fit technique (Fig. 4.2).

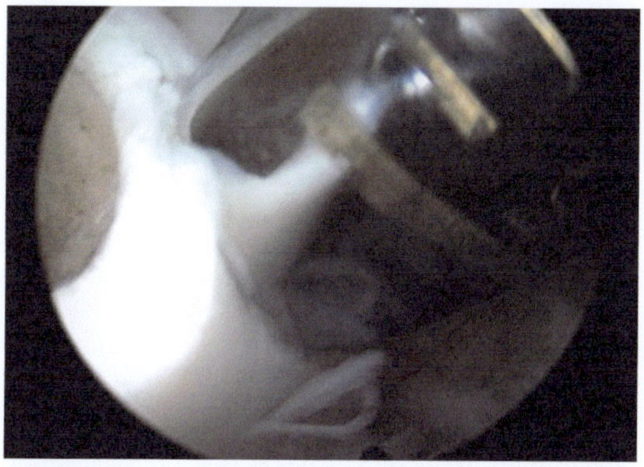

Fig. 4.1 Harvesting the osteochondral defect by means of a gouge

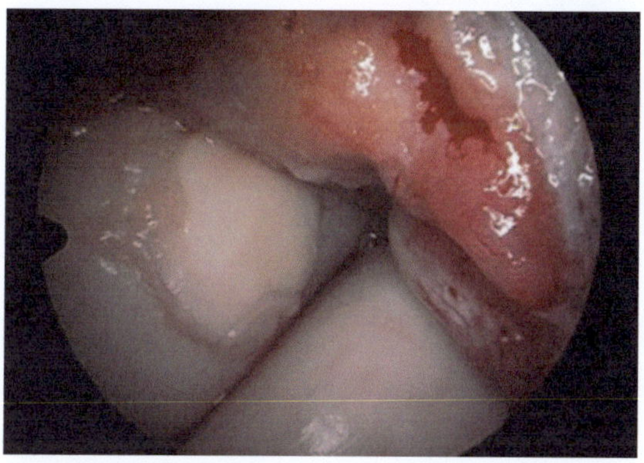

Fig. 4.2 Condition after inserting an OATS cylinder in the elbow joint

A protrusion of the cylinder or a visible gap formation between the cylinder and the surrounding tissue should be avoided.

This technique presents a sufficient option for the treatment of an OCL in the elbow joint. However, in some cases, persistent pain can occur in the knee joint (donor area). The patient must be informed about this possibility. This technique can lead to good results with excellent clinical scores regarding pain, elbow mobility, and return to sports [2, 6, 17, 27].

Another surgical technique is represented by matrix-induced chondrocyte transplantation (MACT) in combination with cancellous bone grafting [29]. This two-stage technique has the advantage, that harvesting of large areas of autologous cartilage is not necessary.

After arthroscopic removal of a small amount of cartilage from the notch, cartilage cells are isolated and cultivated on a 3D scaffold. In a second surgery, this scaffold is implanted into the defect using an open surgical approach [29, 30] (approach similar to the OATS technique) after reconstruction of the defect of the subchondral bone by autologous or allogenic cancellous bone. After fixation of the scaffold using resorbable sutures, the graft has sufficient stability to ensure safe healing. Preliminary data of this technique showed promising results. However, long-term studies regarding this technique in the elbow joint do not exist and have to be performed in the future.

4.6.5 Our Own Technique

The indication for surgical treatment of an osteochondral lesion in the elbow depends on the grade of the OCL regarding the classification of Dipaola et al. Grade III° and IV° lesions in combination with a closed growth plate are indications for surgical treatment. In these cases, autologous osteochondral transfer or MACT with subchondral bone grafting is performed. In low-grade lesions (I°–II°) with closed growth plates, arthroscopic debridement is the treatment of choice.

If the growth plates are still open, a conservative treatment is initiated and the patient is advised to avoid load bearing of the joint but to maintain mobility until complete healing of the defect is achieved and proven by MRI. However, in the presence of a loose fragment that causes mechanical locking of the joint, surgical fragment fixation should be performed, and if this is not possible, an arthroscopic fragment resection should be done. If complaints persist postoperatively, an osteochondral transplantation should be discussed after the closure of the growth plate.

4.7 Summary

The osteochondral lesion of the capitulum mainly affects adolescents who participate in throwing sports or gymnastics.

The etiology of osteochondral lesions is presumably multifactorial. However, in the elbow, it is mainly caused by repetitive microtraumata.

Stable lesions with open growth plates should be treated by conservative therapy.

In unstable lesions, especially after growth plates are closed, the operative treatment is the therapy of choice. Several surgical procedures are described and can be used in the treatment of osteochondral lesions.

The transfer of an (autologous) cartilage–bone cylinder, as well as the MACT with subchondral bone grafting, is a possible treatment option that should be considered dependent on the extent of the defect to sufficiently replace both the damaged cartilage and bone.

Long-term studies after osteochondral transplantation show superior clinical and radiological results compared to other surgical techniques.

References

1. Ruchelsman DE, Hall MP, Youm T. Osteochondritis dissecans of the capitellum: current concepts. J Am Acad Orthop Surg. 2010;18:557–67.
2. Vogt S, Siebenlist S, Hensler D, et al. Osteochondral transplantation in the elbow leads to good clinical and radiologic long-term results: an 8- to 14-year follow-up examination. Am J Sports Med. 2011;39:2619–25.
3. Mihara K, Tsutsui H, Nishinaka N, Yamaguchi K. Nonoperative treatment for osteochondritis dissecans of the capitellum. Am J Sports Med. 2009;37:298–304.
4. Mihara K, Suzuki K, Makiuchi D, Nishinaka N, Yamaguchi K, Tsutsui H. Surgical treatment for osteochondritis dissecans of the humeral capitellum. J Shoulder Elb Surg. 2010;19:31–7.
5. Takeda H, Watarai K, Matsushita T, Saito T, Terashima Y. A surgical treatment for unstable osteochondritis dissecans lesions of the humeral capitellum in adolescent baseball players. Am J Sports Med. 2002;30:713–7.
6. Yamamoto Y, Ishibashi Y, Tsuda E, Sato H, Toh S. Osteochondral autograft transplantation for osteochondritis dissecans of the elbow in juvenile baseball players: minimum 2-year follow-up. Am J Sports Med. 2006;34:714–20.
7. Laurent LE, Lindstrom BL. Osteochondrosis of the capitulum humeri: Panner's disease. Acta Orthop Scand. 1956;26:111–9.
8. Panner H. An affection of the capitulum humeri resembling Calvé-Perthes' disease of the hip. Acta Radiol. 1927;10:234–42.
9. Kobayashi K, Burton KJ, Rodner C, Smith B, Caputo AE. Lateral compression injuries in the pediatric elbow: Panner's disease and osteochondritis dissecans of the capitellum. J Am Acad Orthop Surg. 2004;12:246–54.
10. König F. Über freie Körper in den Gelenken. Dtsch Z Chir. 1888;27:90–109.
11. Edmonds EW, Polousky J. A review of knowledge in osteochondritis dissecans: 123 years of minimal evolution from König to the ROCK Study Group. Clin Orthop Relat Res. 2013;471:1118–26.
12. Bradley JP, Petrie RS. Osteochondritis dissecans of the humeral capitellum. Diagnosis and treatment. Clin Sports Med. 2001;20:565–90.
13. Kusumi T, Ishibashi Y, Tsuda E, et al. Osteochondritis dissecans of the elbow: histopathological assessment of the articular cartilage and subchondral bone with emphasis on their damage and repair. Pathol Int. 2006;56:604–12.
14. Schenck RC, Athanasiou KA, Constantinides G, Gomez E. A biomechanical analysis of articular cartilage of the human elbow and a potential relationship to osteochondritis dissecans. Clin Orthop Relat Res. 1994;(299):305–12.
15. Yadao MA, Field LD, Savoie FH. Osteochondritis dissecans of the elbow. Instr Course Lect. 2004;53:599–606.
16. Klingele KE, Kocher MS. Little league elbow: valgus overload injury in the paediatric athlete. Sports Med. 2002;32:1005–15.
17. Ansah P, Vogt S, Ueblacker P, Martinek V, Woertler K, Imhoff AB. Chondral transplantation to treat osteochondral lesions in the elbow. J Bone Joint Surg. 2007;89:2188–94.
18. Ruch DS, Cory JW, Poehling GG. The arthroscopic management of osteochondritis dissecans of the adolescent elbow. Arthroscopy. 1998;14:797–803.
19. Takahara M, Mura N, Sasaki J, Harada M, Ogino T. Classification, treatment, and outcome of osteochondritis dissecans of the humeral capitellum. J Bone Joint Surg Am. 2007;89:1205–14.
20. Dipaola JD, Nelson DW, Colville MR. Characterizing osteochondral lesions by magnetic resonance imaging. Arthroscopy. 1991;7:101–4.
21. Nelson DW, DiPaola J, Colville M, Schmidgall J. Osteochondritis dissecans of the talus and knee: prospective comparison of MR and arthroscopic classifications. J Comput Assist Tomogr. 1990;14:804–8.
22. Takahara M, Ogino T, Fukushima S, Tsuchida H, Kaneda K. Nonoperative treatment of osteochondritis dissecans of the humeral capitellum. Am J Sports Med. 1999;27:728–32.
23. Mitsunaga MM, Adishian DA, Bianco AJ. Osteochondritis dissecans of the capitellum. J Trauma. 1982;22:53–5.
24. Brownlow HC, O'Connor-Read LM, Perko M. Arthroscopic treatment of osteochondritis dissecans of the capitellum. Knee Surg Sports Traumatol Arthrosc. 2006;14:198–202.

25. Rahusen FTG, Brinkman J-M, Eygendaal D. Results of arthroscopic debridement for osteochondritis dissecans of the elbow. Br J Sports Med. 2006;40:966–9.
26. Schoch B, Wolf BR. Osteochondritis dissecans of the capitellum: minimum 1-year follow-up after arthroscopic debridement. Arthroscopy. 2010;26:1469–73.
27. Shimada K, Yoshida T, Nakata K, Hamada M, Akita S. Reconstruction with an osteochondral autograft for advanced osteochondritis dissecans of the elbow. Clin Orthop Relat Res. 2005;(435):140–7.
28. Bauer M, Jonsson K, Josefsson PO, Lindén B. Osteochondritis dissecans of the elbow. A long-term followup study. Clin Orthop Relat Res. 1992;(284):156–60.
29. Kircher J. Autologous chondrocyte implantation for post-traumatic cartilage defect of capitulum humeri. J Shoulder Elbow Surg. 2016;25(7):e213–6.
30. Ebert JR, Fallon M, Wood DJ, Janes GC. A prospective clinical and radiological evaluation at 5 years after arthroscopic matrix-induced autologous chondrocyte implantation. Am J Sports Med. 2017;45(1):59–69.

Loose Bodies

5

Christian Gerhardt and Markus Scheibel

Contents

5.1 Introduction

The removal of loose bodies from the elbow is an absolute indication of an arthroscopic procedure. However, it is essential to know the neurovascular anatomy of the elbow as well as the adequate placement of the arthroscopic portals to avoid complications. After the knee joint, the elbow joint is the second most common location of loose bodies. [1, 2].

Loose bodies in the elbow joint can arise due to various causes, whereby osteoarthritis is certainly one of the most common causes [1].

5.2 Pathology

In principle, different etiologies that are responsible for the development of loose bodies can be differentiated; however, the cause lies in struc-

C. Gerhardt (✉)
Department for Trauma and Hand Surgery, ViDia Kliniken Karlsruhe, Karlsruhe, Germany
e-mail: Christian.gerhardt@vincentius-ka.de

M. Scheibel
Department of Shoulder and Elbow Surgery, Schulthess Klinik, Zürich, Switzerland
e-mail: scheibel.info@kws.ch

A. B. Imhoff, A. Lenich (eds.), *Elbow Arthroscopy and Minimal Invasive Surgery*,
https://doi.org/10.1007/978-3-031-75611-5_5

tures that line the joint. James Milgram described a classification that basically includes three causes [3]:

- In the context of proliferative changes of the synovium, for example, synovial osteochondromatosis
- Osteochondral fragments in situ, for example, caused by osteochondrosis dissecans or due to a traumatic genesis
- Loss of integrity of the articular surfaces, for example, degenerative arthritis or avascular necrosis

Based on this differentiation and in cases of an unknown etiology, it is necessary to take biopsies from the synovium to examine them for possible multifocal chondral or osteochondral metaplastic proliferation [4].

5.3 Indication

The indication for the arthroscopic removal of loose bodies includes symptomatic patients with recurrent pain and blockage symptoms. If possible, the surgeon should find out the cause, localization, and etiology of the loose bodies, as the clinical outcome is often determined by the underlying disease and not just by the removal of the loose bodies.

5.3.1 Medical History

A careful medical history is essential to detect possible causes of the loose bodies. The main symptom of loose bodies is pain. In addition, mechanical problems such as blockages or crepitations may occur. Either due to entrapment phenomena or reactive synovitis, restriction of the range of motion, especially extension, is possible.

Previous traumas such as fractures, falls, or dislocations should be evaluated and documented. However, even repetitive microtrauma, for example, in overhead athletes or weightlifters can cause changes that lead to loose bodies. In addition, previous operations, in particular neurolysis or transposition of the ulnar nerve, should be evaluated. Especially, after a transposition, the nerve should be exposed to avoid injury when establishing an arthroscopic portal.

5.3.2 Clinical Evaluation

The clinical evaluation begins with the inspection, which is often inconspicuous. However, in some cases, a discreet joint effusion may be apparent.

Tenderness is occasionally reported in the area of the loose body. The assessment of the range of motion is essential in comparison to the opposite side. If there is a painful restriction of movement, a differentiation must be made to evaluate if the pain occurs during the movement or at the end of the movement. Occasionally, crepitus can be palpated.

Of course, the clinical examination to assess the underlying pathology must be carried out completely and should include stability tests as well as a survey of the neurovascular status.

5.3.3 Diagnostic Imaging

5.3.3.1 Conventional X-Ray

The first step in imaging is the conventional X-ray in two views: anteroposterior (a.p.) and lateral (Fig. 5.1). A distinction can already be made between congenital and acquired loose bodies. Furthermore, statements can be made on the degenerative state of the joint, the localization of radiopaque joint bodies, and proof of injuries in case of acute trauma.

However, due to the complex anatomy of the elbow, cross-sectional image diagnostics (CT and MRI) are necessary to validate and characterize the location, obtain information on the consistency and mobility of the loose bodies, and give more detailed information about the etiology of the loose bodies.

5.3.3.2 Cross-Sectional Imaging

For various reasons, the MRI examination of the elbow joint has now become the diagnostic tool of choice (Fig. 5.2). On the one hand, it decreases

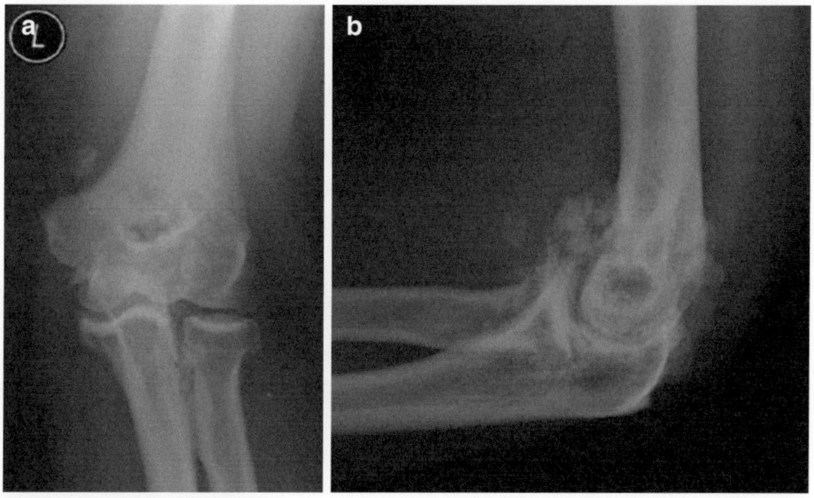

Fig. 5.1 Conventional X-ray images of left elbow in two planes with early cubital osteoarthritis and free loose bodies

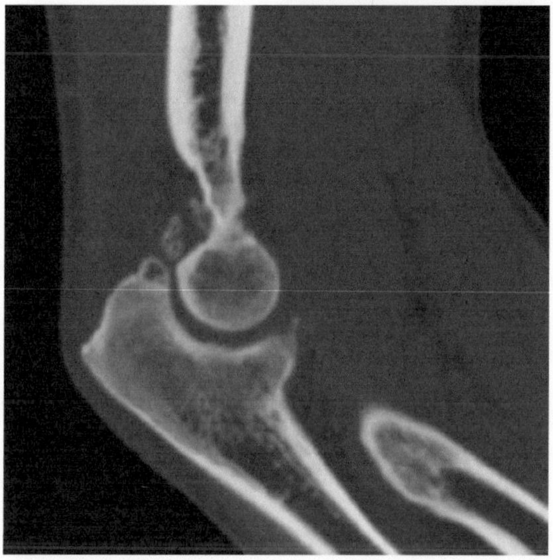

Fig. 5.2 CT image with free joint loose bodies, especially in the olecranon fossa

the exposure to radiation in comparison to CT; on the other hand, the MRI has more advantages, which include the good presentation of the soft-tissue structures such as non-radiopaque loose bodies, ligamentous structures, or cartilage surfaces. Dubberley et al. found a high sensitivity but low specificity for MRI and CT in the detection of loose bodies in the elbow [5] in their study that included 26 patients.

Preoperative imaging is useful for localization and determining the number of loose bodies, to plan the arthroscopic accessibility and to be able to remove them completely. Typically, the loose bodies are located in the coronoid fossa, olecranon fossa, or radial recess. Nevertheless, all other compartments, for example, the ulnar recess, should be also assessed, as loose bodies can be located in any compartment or can migrate to it.

5.4 Principle of Operation/Instruments

Nowadays, the arthroscopic intervention for the removal of loose bodies from the elbow joint is well established. Similar to other joints, careful inspection of different joint compartments is essential, not only to remove the loose bodies but also to be able to detect and treat any other accompanying pathologies. If possible, the underlying pathology should be determined, and the etiology should be detected. In fact, the effective therapy of the primary pathology makes more sense than the sole removal of the loose bodies [1, 6].

As a rule, the standard instruments of the arthroscopy are sufficient. This includes an inlet cannula, a trocar, a 30-degree lens, at least two switching sticks, grasping forceps, and curved, sharp clamps. An electrothermal instrument and a shaver are very helpful.

Depending on the underlying pathology, additional instruments such as small chisels, curettes, or instruments for microfracture may be needed.

5.5 Preparation for Surgery

The positioning of the patient and the portals used are described in Chap. 3.

The patient can be positioned in either a lateral or prone position. The lateral position has various advantages in terms of simplicity of positioning and the accessibility of the airway to anesthesia. However, in obese patients, the abdominal soft tissue may limit the mobility of the instruments in the lateral position, which is why the prone position may be preferred in some of the procedures.

General anesthesia is usually sufficient for the removal of loose bodies. However, in the case of accompanying stiff elbow or other intra-articular pathologies, it is preferred to insert an axillary or interscalenous catheter to ease the postoperative pain therapy.

5.6 Surgical Technique

After positioning the patient and application of the tourniquet, the affected extremity is sterilized and covered. Then, the bony landmarks are marked with a sterile marker (Fig. 5.3).

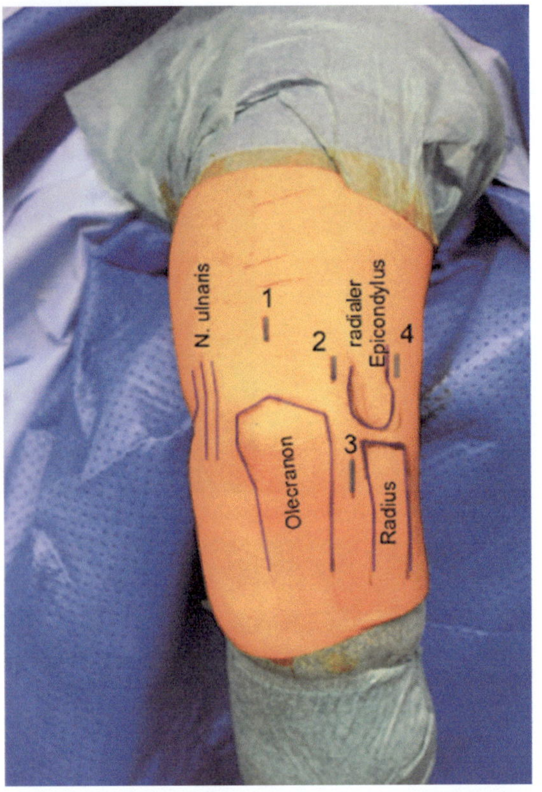

Fig. 5.3 Marking of the bony landmarks; this takes place after the patient has been positioned, 1—posterior transtendinous (triceps) portal, 2—high posteroradial portal, 3—deep posteroradial portal in the soft spot, 4—anteroradial portal

To achieve safe arthroscopic access to the joint, distension of the joint is needed, and this is achieved through injection of about 20–30 mL of sterile saline solution through the "soft-spot portal" or directly into the olecranon fossa [7, 8].

In our own approach, an anterolateral portal is created, and the joint is punctured with the beveled cannula (Fig. 5.4). In this way, safe access to the ventral compartment is established even with increasing soft-tissue swelling. However, in arthrofibrotic joints, the water inflow to the posterior compartment may be restricted, so that the inflow must be changed afterward.

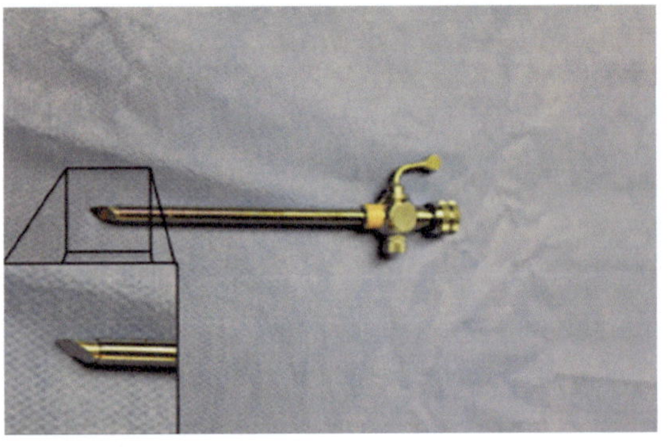

Fig. 5.4 Angled inlet cannula

Now, a posterolateral portal is established slightly proximal to the tip of the olecranon, lateral to the triceps tendon, and a switching stick is inserted and directed to the olecranon fossa.

The trocar is introduced into the posterior compartment through this portal and the optic is then connected. The posterior compartment is now viewed, exposing the ulnar recess, the tip of the olecranon, and the olecranon fossa (Fig. 5.5).

For evaluation of a possible instability and for the removal of loose bodies, a posterior, transtendinous portal is created through the triceps tendon. The loose bodies can be removed with grasping forceps with slightly rotatory movements.

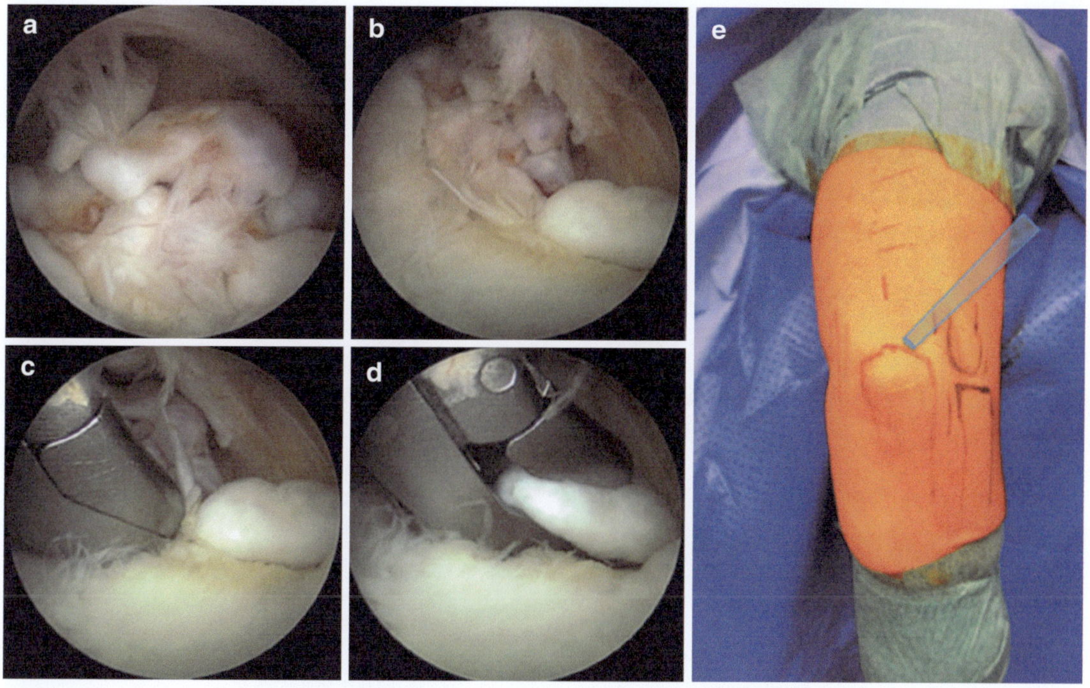

Fig. 5.5 Arthroscopic images showing multiple free joint loose bodies in the olecranon fossa; (**a**, **b**) the fossa is completely relocated by several free joint bodies; (**c**, **d**) after posterior, transtendinous portals, these can be removed with a rongeur; (**e**) positioning the optics in the high posteroradial portal

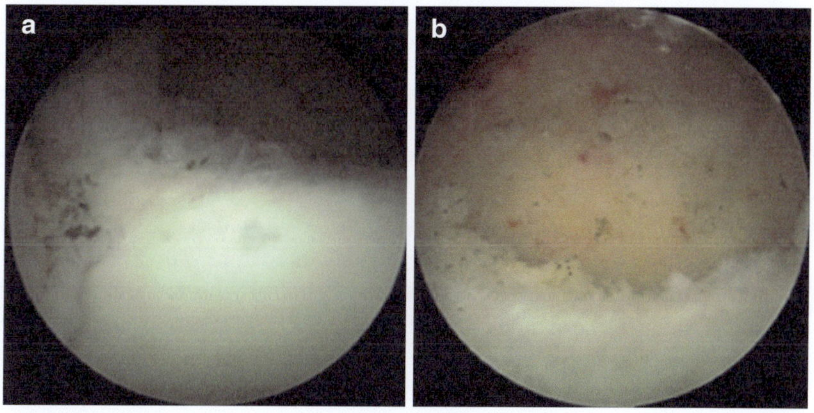

Fig. 5.6 After removal of the free joint loose bodies and debridement or resection of osteophytes in early cubital osteoarthritis, the olecranon fossa is free

It is important to ensure that the portal is large enough to avoid losing the loose bodies in the soft tissues (Fig. 5.6). It is necessary to carefully spread the portal with a clamp or scissors. Adherent loose bodies should be released beforehand. If the loose body is significantly larger than the portal size, it must be removed piece by piece. An alternative is to reduce its size with a shaver or acromionizer until it can be easily removed. Particularly in the case of loose bodies in the ulnar recess, the proximity of the ulnar nerve below the joint capsule must be considered. To keep the soft tissues away, it may be necessary to create a posteroradial portal and to hold the soft tissue away with a switching stick or a retractor. Another possibility is to "strike out" the ulnar recess from distal to proximal. In this way, small and deep-lying loose bodies can also be shifted into the olecranon fossa.

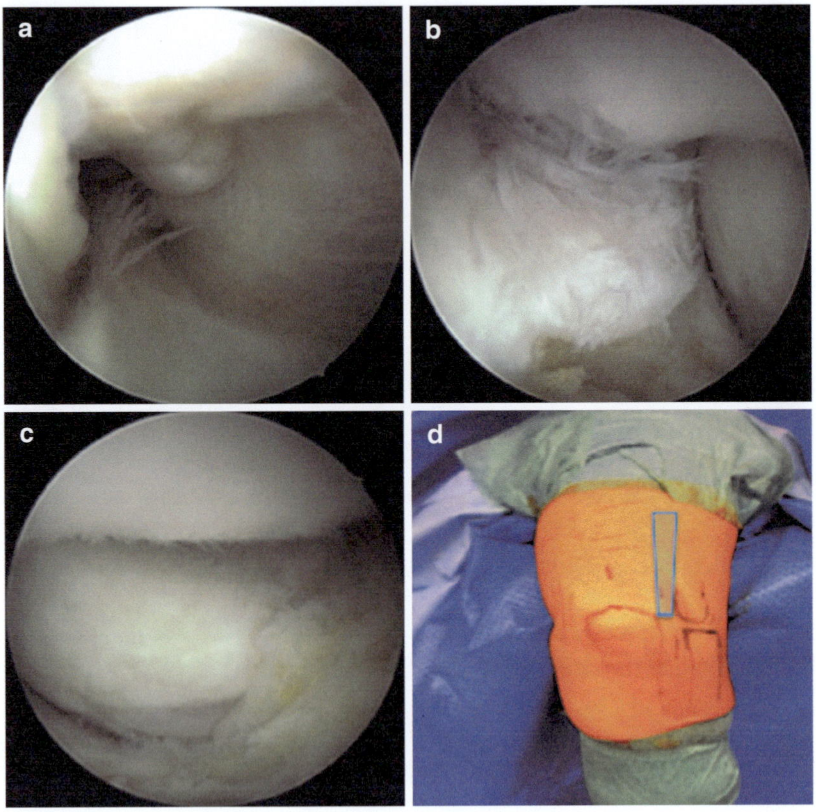

Fig. 5.7 (**a**) The camera is positioned in the radial recess and advanced distally until the radial head is visible (**b**, **c**). (**d**) Positioning of the camera in the high posteroradial portal

The next step is to inspect the radial recess. The arthroscope is inserted along the radial humeroulnar joint space. In the arthritic joints or in posttraumatic conditions, the joint can be obstructed by osteophytes or hypertrophic synovitis.

Insertion of the optic in the posterior, transtendinous portal is done to enable direct visualization of the radial recess, this can be aided by forward pushing of the switching stick. The radial recess is now carefully viewed, and a portal is created in the soft spot under direct view. In some cases, the resection of a hypertrophic synovitis or a prominent posterior plica is necessary. Here also, careful attention must be given to loose bodies, accompanying instability, or the presence of chondral lesions (Fig. 5.7).

The switching stick is inserted through the anterioradial inlet cannula, which is then removed, and the trocar is inserted and viewed in the ventral compartment (Fig. 5.8). The loose bodies are often located in the coronoid fossa. The medial recess, the coronoid process, the trochlea, the ventral capsule, the capitulum, the radial head, and, in some cases, the radial recess can be inspected from medial to lateral.

In the next step, an anteromedial portal should be established. For this purpose, the arthroscope should be positioned in the area that is needed the most for the rest of the procedure. To achieve this, the O'Driscoll technique is performed, and a switching stick can be pushed through the capsule, flexors, and subcutaneous tissue to make the skin incision against the desired area [6]. Alternatively, this portal can be created approx. 2 cm proximal to the medial humeral epicondyle and ventral to the intermuscular septum using the outside-in technique. It must be ensured that only one skin incision is made, and the deeper tissue parts should be bluntly perforated to avoid damaging of the neurovascular structures. After finishing the procedure as removal of the loose bodies or partial synovectomy, the joint must be inspected from the medial side to detect and assess radially located pathologies. The use of a switching stick is ideal for this purpose.

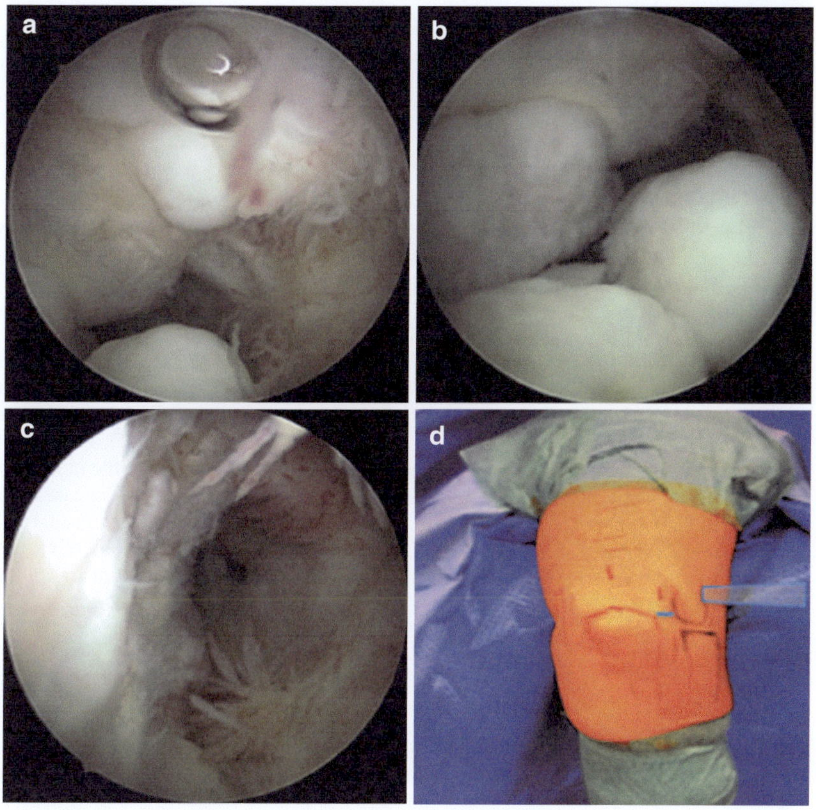

Fig. 5.8 The anterior compartment is inspected through the anteroradial portal. (**a**) Several free joint bodies anteriorly; (**b**) the coronoid process shows osteophytes in early osteoarthritis; (**c**) after removal of the free joint bodies, reactive hypertrophic synovitis becomes apparent; (**d**) Positioning the optics in the high anteroradial portal

After removing the instruments, the wound is closed, and a compression bandage is applied.

5.6.1 Complications

The most feared complication is nerve injuries, which are rare and usually transient. In the literature, the incidence is about 0–14% [9–12]. Although these tend to occur in more complex procedures, lesions of the ulnar nerve, the median nerve, and the deep branch of the radial nerve have been described.

5.6.2 Results

Clasper et al. described in their retrospective evaluation the results of 57 arthroscopies of the elbow joint ($n = 54$ patients), the patients were subjected to arthroscopic intervention if the presence of loose bodies was suspected [1]. About 80% of the patients have benefited from the procedure, especially those who had loose bodies.

O'Driscoll et al. reported the results of 24 elbow arthroscopies in which loose bodies were removed in 18 cases [6]. Patients without any other pathology have benefited the most from the intervention, whereas the sole removal of loose bodies without addressing possible accompanying pathologies (e.g., early osteoarthritis) generally leads to poorer results.

5.7 Postoperative Measures

Immobilization is not necessary if only loose bodies are removed. A pain-adapted passive and active mobilization is possible from the first postoperative day. After the removal of the stitches and achieving free mobility, the loading of the joint can be increased gradually.

Changes and adjustments of the postoperative measures depend on the underlying pathology or the performed operative therapy.

References

1. Clasper JC, Carr AJ. Arthroscopy of the elbow for loose bodies. Ann R Coll Surg Engl. 2001;83:34–6.
2. Phemister DB. The causes and changes in loose bodies arising from the articular surface of the joint. J Bone Joint Surg. 1924;6:278–315.
3. Milgram JW. The classification of loose bodies in human joints. Clin Orthop Relat Res. 1977;(124):282–91.
4. Milgram JW. Synovial osteochondromatosis: a histopathological study of thirty cases. J Bone Joint Surg Am. 1977;59:792–801.
5. Dubberley JH, Faber KJ, Patterson SD. The detection of loose bodies in the elbow. J Bone Joint Surg. 2005;87(5):684–6.
6. O'Driscoll SW, Morrey BF. Arthroscopy of the elbow. Diagnostic and therapeutic benefits and hazards. J Bone Joint Surg Am. 1992;74:84–94.
7. Hackl M, Lappen S, Burkhart KJ, et al. Elbow positioning and joint insufflation substantially influence median and radial nerve locations. Clin Orthop Relat Res. 2015;473:3627–34.
8. Miller CD, Jobe CM, Wright MH. Neuroanatomy in elbow arthroscopy. J Shoulder Elb Surg. 1995;4:168–74.
9. Kelly EW, Morrey BF, O'Driscoll SW. Complications of elbow arthroscopy. J Bone Joint Surg Am. 2001;83-A:25–34.
10. Lynch GJ, Meyers JF, Whipple TL, Caspari RB. Neurovascular anatomy and elbow arthroscopy: inherent risks. Arthroscopy. 1986;2:190–7.
11. Papilion JD, Neff RS, Shall LM. Compression neuropathy of the radial nerve as a complication of elbow arthroscopy: a case report and review of the literature. Arthroscopy. 1988;4:284–6.
12. Ruch DS, Poehling GG. Anterior interosseus nerve injury following elbow arthroscopy. Arthroscopy. 1997;13:756–8.

Elbow Dislocation

6

Andreas Lenich and Sebastian Siebenlist

Contents

6.1 Introduction

The dislocation of the elbow is the second most common dislocation of large joints. The purely ligamentous dislocations must be differentiated from elbow fracture dislocations. After the reduction, an exact diagnosis must be made to define the extent of damage. Only by an accurate diagnostic the indication for either conservative or surgical treatment can be made. The arthroscopy (ASK) of the elbow joint

A. Lenich (✉)
ZEST – Zentrum for Elbow and Shoulder Therapy, Munich, Germany

S. Siebenlist
Department of Orthopaedic Sports Medicine, Klinikum Rechts der Isar, Technical University of Munich, Munich, Germany
e-mail: Sebastian.Siebenlist@tum.de

A. B. Imhoff, A. Lenich (eds.), *Elbow Arthroscopy and Minimal Invasive Surgery*,
https://doi.org/10.1007/978-3-031-75611-5_6

can be used both as a diagnostic measure as well as a therapeutic measure, it is therefore considered as an important tool in the treatment of different pathologies [1]. Recently, arthroscopy has been considered as an additive diagnostic tool that become increasingly popular [2, 3].

6.2 Pathology

6.2.1 Ligamentous Elbow Dislocation

The purely ligamentous dislocation occurs primarily in young patients, distinguished and classified according to the direction of dislocation. In 80% of the cases, the directions of dislocations are commonly the dorsal or dorsoradial dislocation. Less common are the ulnar and ventral dislocation directions (about 20%). In high-speed traumas, the divergent dislocation is observed (<1%). In ligamentous elbow dislocation, the capsuloligamentous structures and cartilage are commonly injured; also, it is not uncommon to see muscle injuries [4].

6.2.2 Elbow Dislocation with Intraarticular Fractures

The accompanying fractures as part of elbow dislocations are usually found in high-speed trauma or patients aged 50 or more. The fractures are dependent on the direction of dislocation and the structures are affected in this descending order:

1. Torn ligaments.
2. Fracture of the radius head.
3. Fracture of the coronoid process.
4. Fracture of the olecranon.

6.3 Diagnosis

6.3.1 History

A medical history to evaluate the accident and to assess the trauma is very important. Paresthesia in the area of supply of the radial, median, and ulnar nerves should be asked and documented.

6.3.2 Clinical Evaluation

After a dislocation has taken place and as part of the clinical investigation, both the elbow joint as well as the wrist joint must be evaluated accordingly. After the inspection of the joint contour and position, the pulse (radial and ulnar arteries) must be checked. The sensation and motor skills of the nerves supplying the forearm (radial, median, and ulnar nerves) must be documented.

The passive and active range of motion of the elbow and wrist must be documented. The varus and valgus stress tests of the elbow show potential instability. The stability of the distal radioulnar joint should be tested dorsally and ventrally.

6.3.3 Diagnostic Imaging

6.3.3.1 Sonography

The sonography of the elbow enables the dynamic visualization of muscular and ligamentous injuries. The stability of the collateral ligaments in the varus and valgus stress test, bleeding into the joint capsule and muscles can also be documented by sonography.

6.3.3.2 Conventional X-Ray Diagnostics

The X-ray of the elbow joint in anteroposterior (a.p.) and lateral views is the golden standard. In addition, a radius head view can be also performed.

The X-ray pictures after reduction can indicate joint instability:

- "delta sign": asymmetrical joint line in the AP image due to a medial or lateral instability or a coronoid fracture.
- "drop sign": increased ulnohumeral distance >3 mm in the lateral image as a sign of persistent rotational instability [5].
- "Stoeren Line": dorsal shifting of the radius/capitulum axis.
- "Osborne-Cotterill Lesion": dorsal bony impression of the capitulum as a sign of the previous dislocation of the radial head behind the capitulum ("Hill Sachs Impression" of the elbow; [6]).

6.3.3.3 CT and MRI Diagnostic

A CT examination of the elbow joint is indicated if there is suspicion of fracture dislocation and free loose bodies to precisely localize and classify them preoperatively.

The ligament and muscular damage can be evaluated using an MRI. Incongruities of joint surfaces caused by cartilage fragments and soft tissue interpositions can also be diagnosed by the MRI.

If possible, the examination must be carried out with nearly full extension of the elbow. This is the only way to reliably assess the incongruences and ligament injuries, as the joint partners only subluxate in the near extension position due to the lack of active muscular guidance [6].

6.4 Indication for the Arthroscopy

If there is suspicion of free loose bodies and cartilage damage, arthroscopy is indicated. In the case of slightly displaced fractures, an arthroscopic-assisted fracture treatment may be indicated. In the case of chronic elbow disease, diagnostic arthroscopy and stability tests of the individual capsular ligament structures are indicated [7].

6.5 Operation Principle/Instruments

- Standard arthroscopic elbow instruments (Chap. 3).
- Kirschner wires and cannulated headless screws (HCS = headless compression screws) for fracture management (Chap. 12).

6.6 Preparation for Surgery

- Using a tourniquet is beneficial, but not required.
- Positioning on the contralateral side.
- Tourniquet to control bleeding, using a flexible arm holder (e.g., Trimano).
- Skin disinfection and sterile covering, marking of the palpable anatomical structures and all approaches to the elbow joint (Chap. 3).
- Team time-out.

6.7 Surgical Technique

- Puncture and filling of the joint after aspiration with irrigation fluid.
- Anterolateral portal for the irrigation cannula. Dorsal aspects of the joint—ulnar recess, radial recess, and olecranon fossa are inspected (Figs. 6.1, 6.2, 6.3, 6.4, 6.5, 6.6, 6.7, 6.8, and 6.9).
- Dorsal portal closure and change to ventral.
- Wound closure subcutaneously and intracutaneously with absorbable sutures.

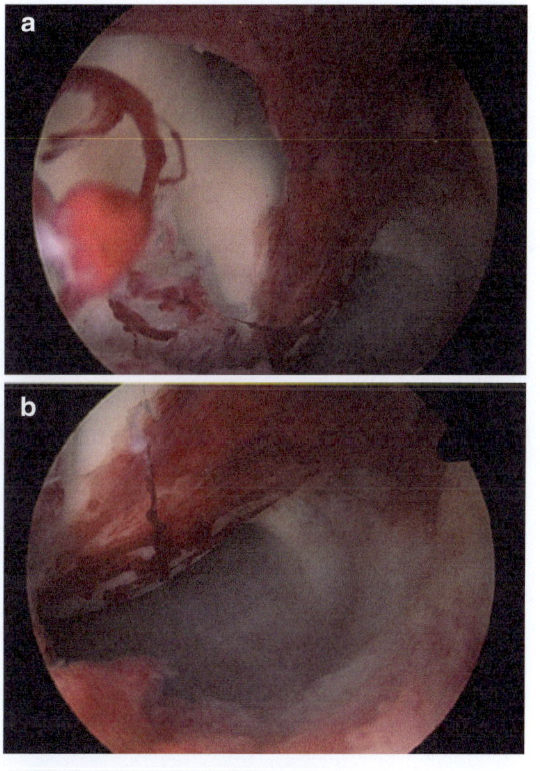

Fig. 6.1 The arthroscopic view of the radial recess (**a**) and ulnar recess (**b**) is difficult after a dislocation due to hematoma formation and tiny loose bodies. These can be removed with the shaver and grasping forceps

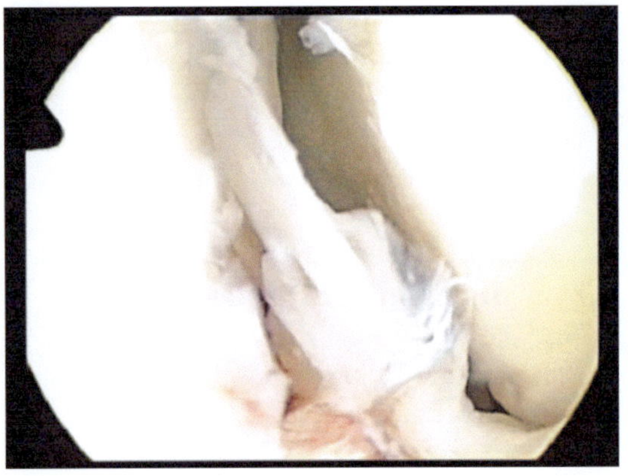

Fig. 6.2 Cartilage fragment in the humeroulnar joint. During the arthroscopic tour, cartilage fragments can be identified and removed. This will prevent blockage and restore the joint movement

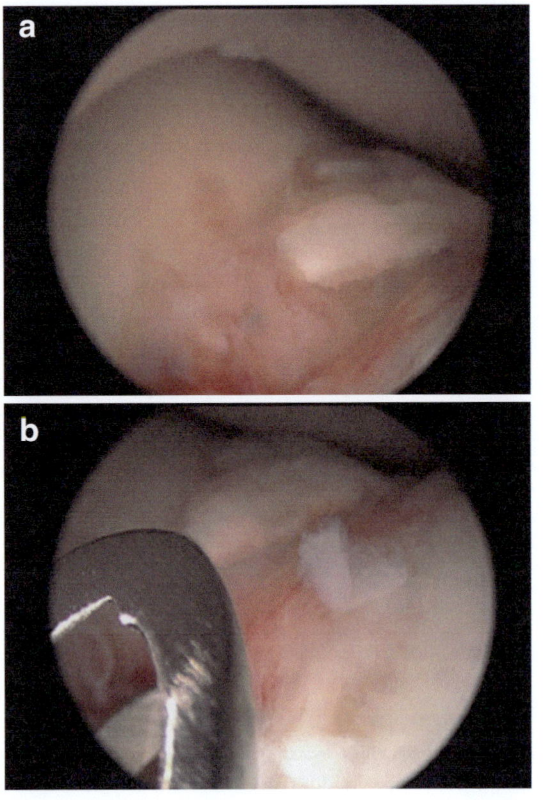

Fig. 6.4 (**a**, **b**) Cartilage defects in the area of the trochlea. (**b**) To prevent the development of a free joint body, this cartilage flake is removed with the Duckbill forceps

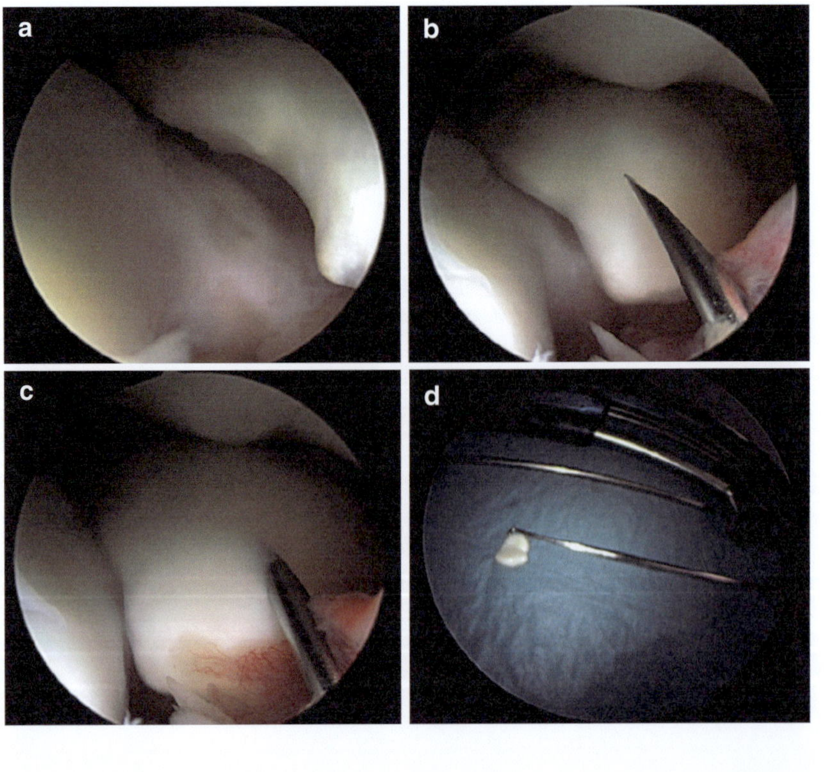

Fig. 6.3 (**a**) Free joint loose body in the humeroulnar joint. (**b**, **c**) In case of very high mobility, this can be fixed with a cannula (needle) to hold the body securely and to prevent it from slipping into inaccessible joint areas. (**d**) The free joint loose body is measured on the operating table and checked for its quality. Stable chips can be refixed. If the pieces of cartilage are smaller than 1 cm^2 or if they are fragmented, replantation is not advisable

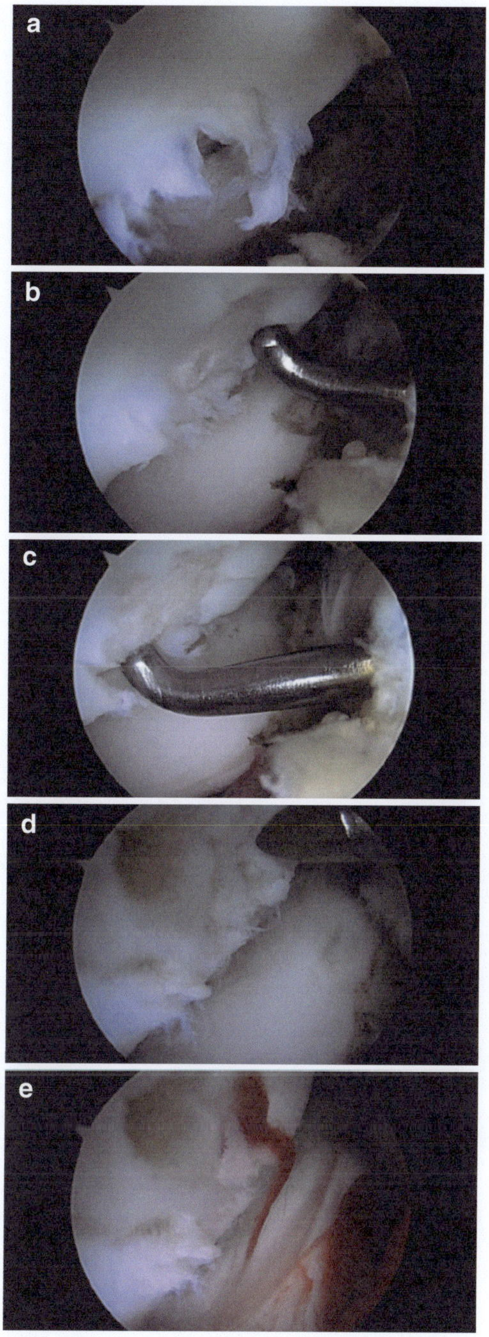

Fig. 6.5 (**a**) Frayed defect on the capitulum. (**b**) After debridement of the loose cartilage, the stability of the defect walls must be checked with the hook. (**c**) To identify fractures, the next step is to examine the stability of the defect base with the probe. (**d**) If the base of the defect is stable, the surface can be microfractured with the microfracture chisel at a distance of 2–3 mm. (**e**) Leaking blood and fat from the bone confirm the success of the maneuver. Sometimes, the flushing fluid pressure must be reduced or stopped to be able to observe this

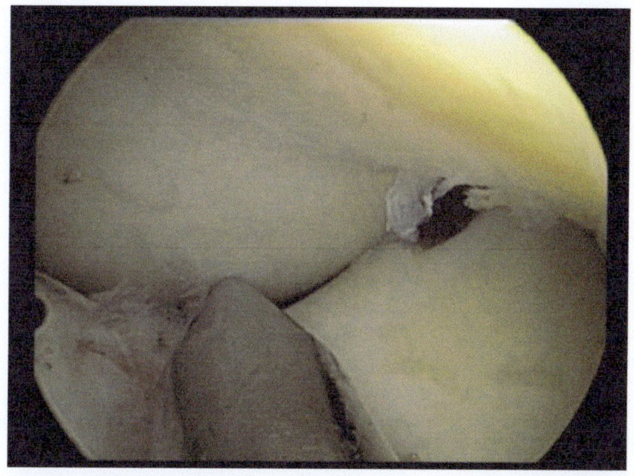

Fig. 6.6 Stability test in the humeroulnar joint with switching stick confirms the lesion of the lateral ulnar collateral ligament (LUCL) and shows a cartilage defect at the tip of the capitulum

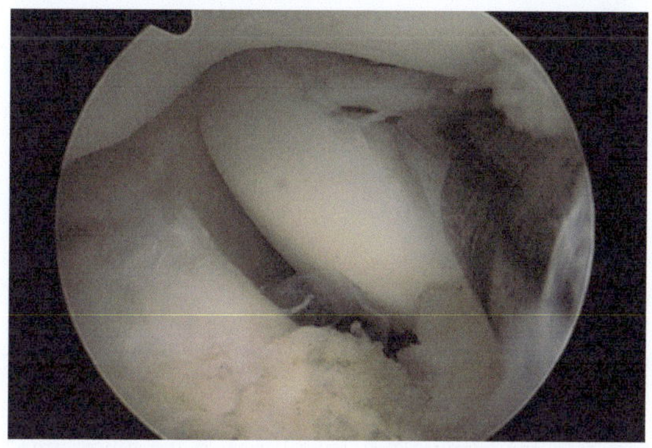

Fig. 6.7 Stability test in the humeroradial joint with the switching stick shows major cartilage damage on the radial head with a stuck cartilage flap

6.7.1 Complications [1–3]

Patients should be informed about the following postoperative complications:

- Remain nerve lesion.
- Temporary nerve affections or paresthesia.
- Reduced mobility of the elbow.
- General surgical complications (e.g., delayed wound healing, fistula formation, infection).

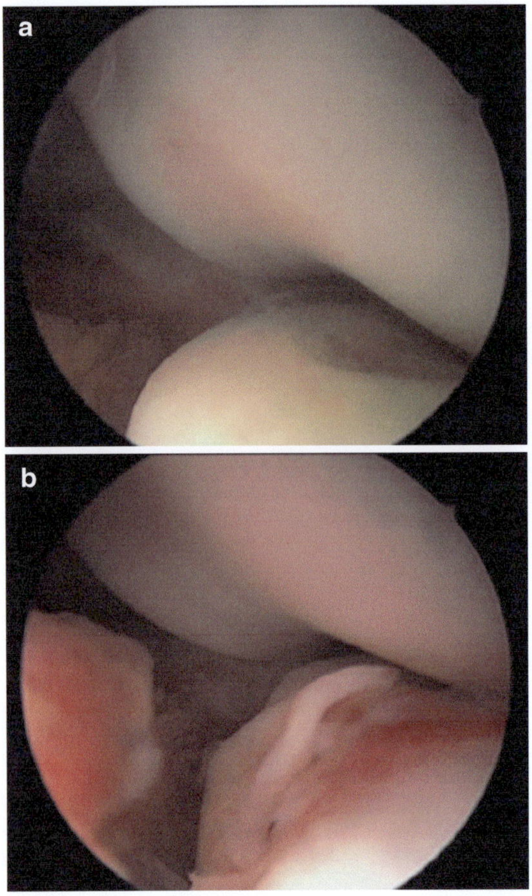

Fig. 6.8 (**a**) View in the ventral part of the elbow joint with uninjured radial head and while the capitulum in the supination position. (**b**) In the same arthroscopic view but in pronation position of the forearm, it shows a fragmented cartilage over an indentation in the head of the radius. It is important to move the joint bodies during a diagnostic tour in order to be able to see all parts safely and to be able to document injuries and, if necessary, treat them

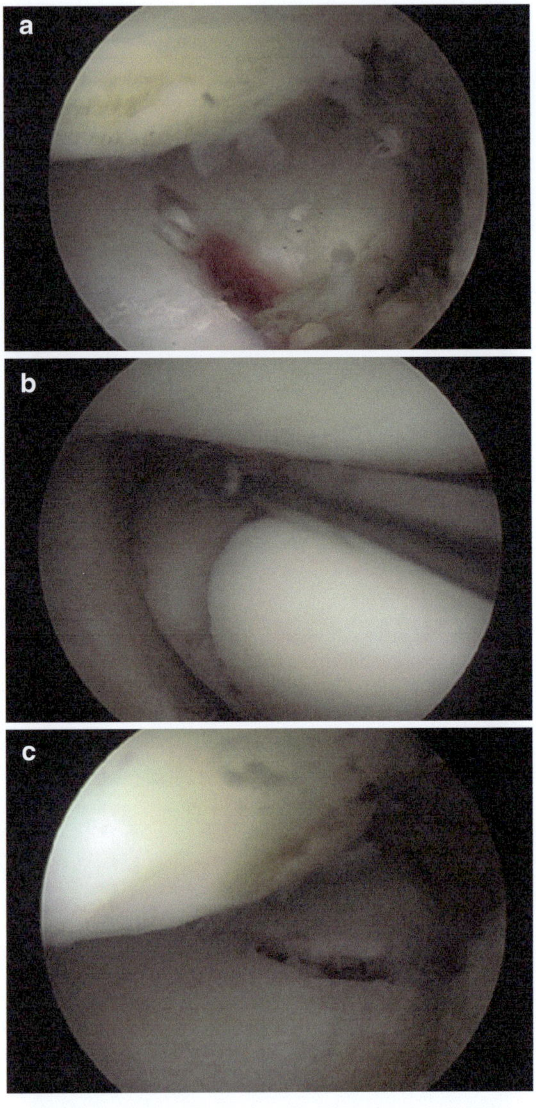

Fig. 6.9 Arthroscopic view of the radial head from dorsoradial. (**a**) Radius head fracture with slight dislocation and fracture hematoma in the fracture gap. (**b**, **c**) Removal of the fragments and the fracture hematoma and reduction of the fracture with the hook. Reduction of the fracture for minimally invasive screw osteosynthesis (7, Chap. 12)

6.8 Postoperative Measures

Follow-up treatment depends on the injury and type of treatment. Thus, a generally applicable scheme for the follow-up treatment of the various possibilities of dislocation cannot be applied and should be determined by the surgeon.

References

1. Vester H, Siebenlist S, Imhoff AB, Lenich A. Arthroscopy of the elbow: diagnostic and therapeutic approaches. Orthopade. 2014;43:943–56.
2. Dexel J, Kasten P. Elbow arthroscopy technique. Arthroscopy. 2013;26:174–80.
3. Hollinger B, Dehlinger F, Franke S. Diagnostic and treatment of elbow instability. Upper Extrem. 2014;9:147–55.
4. Adolfsson LE, Nestorson JO, Scheer JH. Extensive soft tissue lesions in redislocated after simple elbow dislocations. J Shoulder Elb Surg. 2017;26(7):1294–7.
5. Coonrad RW, Roush TF, Major NM, Basamania CJ. The drop sign, a radiographic warning sign of elbow instability. J Shoulder Elb Surg. 2005;14:312–7.
6. Osborne G, Cotterill P. Recurrent dislocation of the elbow. J Bone Joint Surg Br. 1966;48:340–6.
7. Siebenlist S, Biberthaler P. Acute soft tissue injuries of the elbow. Trauma Occup Illn. 2013;17(Suppl 1):132–9.

Radial Instability

7

Christian Schoch and Michael Geyer

Contents

7.1 Etiology

The posterolateral elbow instability can occur due to an isolated varus or hyperextension injury; it can also happen after conservatively treated elbow dislocation.

The posterolateral rotational instability (PLRI) can persist after surgical treatment of macro instability. Chronic instability can also develop without macrotrauma: repetitive microtrauma during sports or occupational exposure can lead to elongation or injury to the posterolateral capsuloligamentous structures, which will end in PLRI.

The incidence of acute elbow instability is 6–13 cases/100,000 inhabitants/year [1]. The number of isolated radial instabilities occurring annually, both acute and chronic, cannot be specified. The authors assume a similarly high number of occult instabilities, which in everyday clinical practice are assigned to "chronic epicondylitis" due to similar symptoms at the tendon insertions [2].

Chronic lateral instability can be relatively discreet in clinical examination and imaging and appear all the more evident under general anesthesia after the loss of muscle tone and, above all, during arthroscopic instability testing.

C. Schoch (✉)
Department for Shoulder and Elbow Surgery, St. Vinzenz Klinik Pfronten, Pfronten, Bavaria, Germany
e-mail: Christian.Schoch@vinzenz-klinik.de

M. Geyer (Retired)
Orthopaedic Department, St. Vinzenz Klinik Pfronten, Pfronten, Bavaria, Germany
e-mail: Michael.Geyer@vinzenz-klinik.de

A. B. Imhoff, A. Lenich (eds.), *Elbow Arthroscopy and Minimal Invasive Surgery*,
https://doi.org/10.1007/978-3-031-75611-5_7

Diagnostic arthroscopy is therefore recommended if the pain in the lateral elbow is unclear.

7.2 Indication

In case of lateral instability, arthroscopy serves on one hand to detect the direction of instability. On the other hand, accompanying pathologies such as chondromalacia or a ruptured plica can also be treated. A stability test using the pivot-shift test, according to O'Driscoll, in an awake patient with a corresponding soft tissue cover and in an anesthetized patient is not always reliably feasible [3]. Sonographic tests on cadaver specimens have now been published, but this is not yet applicable in everyday clinical practice [4].

Radiologically, the PLRI can also be suspected in the biplane X-ray images. The use of an image intensifier with the elbow flexed at 45° with a powerfully supinated forearm can reveal the subluxation if present [5]. After the instability has been verified by an image intensifier, the cartilage damage and other accompanying intraarticular pathologies like instability and lateral elbow pain can be overlooked. In the case of lateral instability, arthroscopy is considered a diagnostic and therapeutic tool for making appropriate therapy decisions.

The stabilization required after a positive diagnosis is done through an open procedure with ligament reconstruction from the triceps tendon or the gracilis tendon. In acute cases, individual working groups report about arthroscopically assisted ligament refixation [6] or ligament tightening [7]. In chronic cases, however, ligament reconstruction with autologous tendon graft is considered the gold standard.

7.3 Operating Principles/Instruments

On the one hand, arthroscopy serves to exclude and treat other accompanying pathologies; on the other hand, it is primarily utilized to diagnose the direction of instability. For this purpose, at least dorsal and dorsolateral arthroscopy with a test instrument (switching stick) must be performed. An attempt is made to evaluate the individual joint partners' stability against each other with a switching stick. For documentation, the absolute extensibility in millimeters and the feeling at the end of the movement is measured.

According to O'Driscoll, instability is classified into three degrees [8]. The accessibility of the switching stick is tested from the dorsal side between the olecranon and humerus at a 90° flexed arm. By pushing with the switching stick, the elbow joint is forced into the ulna's rotatory posterolateral instability in relation to the humerus (PLRI). In unstable joints, dorsal subluxation of the coronoid occurs. If necessary, the switching stick can be pushed from the dorsal side over the coronoid tip or across the joint between the ulna and humerus ("drive-through sign"). The stability of the proximal radioulnar joint (PRUJ) and the pure varus/valgus instability can also be evaluated. In a rotation corresponding to "the pincer grip,“ the radial head's dorsalization against the capitulum can be assessed. In cases of extensive instability, pathognomonic cartilage erosions at the edge of the radius head are easily recognizable arthroscopically. Possible accompanying pathologies such as synovial hypertrophy or chondromalacia can be treated with debridement (Fig. 7.1).

The following instruments are required for the arthroscopic stability test (with a therapeutic option):

- Vacuum mattresses for lateral positioning of the patient.
- Arm holder.
- Tourniquet (optional).
- Sterile skin markers.
- Sterile 20 mL syringe and puncture cannula (for joint filling).
- Scalpel (No. 11).
- Inflow cannula.
- Standard 4 mm arthroscope with 30° optic with trocar, trocar sleeve, and light source.
- Switching stick (4 mm).
- Shaver (e.g., 3.5 mm).
- Sutures for skin closure.

If a lateral ulnar collateral ligament (LUCL) surgery is to be performed, the following instruments are also required:

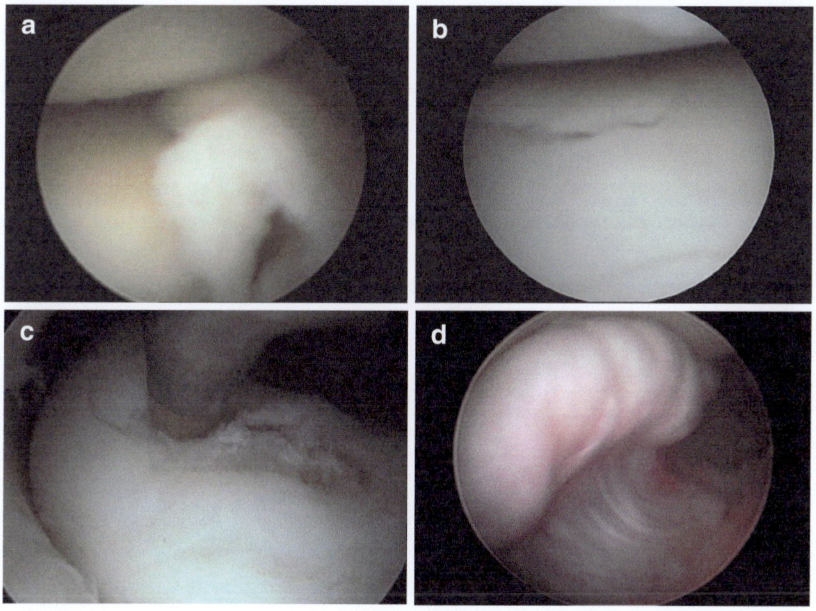

Fig. 7.1 Possible accompanying pathologies: (**a**) plica, (**b**) Cartilage damage of the radial head (pathognomonic on the edge of the radial head), (**c**) Microfracture of central cartilage damage, (**d**) pathognomonic osteophytes in the coronoid fossa

- Arm positioning table.
- Scalpel (No. 20).
- Sharp hooks, Langenbeck hooks, small Hohmann hooks, dissecting scissors.
- Guidewire for over-drilling with a 5-mm drill.
- Biceps button for ulnar fixation (alternatively tenodesis screw).
- 4.75 mm PEEK tenodesis screw (alternatively, e.g., SwiveLock 4.75 mm PEEK) with a suit able screwdriver, 2 × highly stable suture threads (e.g., FibreWire No. 2/FibreLoop), or tape for reinforcement.
- 2.5 mm drill bits (for transosseous sutures, alternatively knot-free anchor).
- Number 0, 1, and 2 absorbable sutures (e.g., Vicryl) for wound closure.

7.4 Operation Preparation

7.4.1 History and Clinical Examination

- Mechanism of the injury, if any.
- Pain history.
- Previous operations (anterior transposition of the ulnar nerve).
- Infiltrations.
- Skin-soft tissue conditions (open wounds, swelling/hematoma, preexisting scars).
- Stability testing while the patient is awake (the patient will complain mostly from apprehension) and under anesthesia (medial/lateral opening of the joint, posterolateral rotational instability, tendency to dislocate).

7.4.2 Imaging

X-rays in two planes represent the basics of imaging diagnostics. Here the "drop sign" or joint incongruences in the anteroposterior (a.p.) plane can be recognized. In chronic instability, magnetic resonance imaging shows the ligaments' injury and possibly the accompanying extensor defect, which can be assessed as a direct sign of instability. The widening of the joint space can also help in the recognition of the respective direction of instability. The dorsal subluxation position of the radial head in the MRI indicates a PLRI. The drop sign is more precise on the MRI and indicates a posterolateral subluxation with an ulna's incongruence to the trochlea. This misalignment of the joint partners can be seen in both sagittal and axial cuts.

An assessment of the extensors is also possible. In case of long-term instability, the clinical problems are not only with the extensors but also degenerations can be detected in the MRI and indicate increased attempts to stabilize the joint with muscles with subsequent tissue fatigue and partial rupture. Likewise, if the disease continues for a long time, osteophytes can be found on the olecranon corresponding to the instability direction [9].

7.5 Surgical Technique

In addition, stability checking is done. Figures 7.2, 7.3, and 7.4 show the three different degrees of the PLRI. Possible accompanying findings such as plica, chondromalacia, and free loose joint bodies (FLB) can be diagnosed and treated (Fig. 7.1).

In rare cases, there is pronounced instability of the proximal radioulnar joint (PRUJ) (Fig. 7.5). The open ligament reconstruction is explained and shown in Fig. 7.6. The procedure is performed under general anesthesia and carried out with the patient lying on his contralateral side. The affected extremity is placed in an arm holder in 90° flexion. Here, the surgeon must ensure that the positioning allows a good range of motion for the operated arm. In particular, there are no obstacles to the flexion of the elbow. Likewise, the consistent padding of the nonoperated arm must be checked (radial nerve). Intravenous antibiotics should be given perioperatively.

After applying a tourniquet with 250 mmHg pressure, sterile washing, and covering, the anatomical landmarks that are important for arthroscopic orientation are marked (tip of the olecranon, radial head, capitulum, trochlea, ulnar nerve). This is followed by joint insufflation with 20–30 mL of NaCl solution via the dorsal "soft-spot portal" and the creation of an anterolateral irrigation portal via a beveled irrigation cannula.

As in any elbow arthroscopy, filling the joint aims to distend the capsule and thus keep the neural structure lying on the capsule away from it. The inlet pressure is built up via the anterolateral irrigation cannula (35–40 mmHg). First, perform a diagnostic tour to detect any accompanying pathologies and treat them accordingly. The superior-posterior portal is used initially as a viewing portal for this purpose. Therefore, the first look is in the olecranon fossa, the ulnar side of the dorsal joint capsule, and the olecranon's tip. To diagnose the instability here, a transtricipital portal can be done so that a switching stick

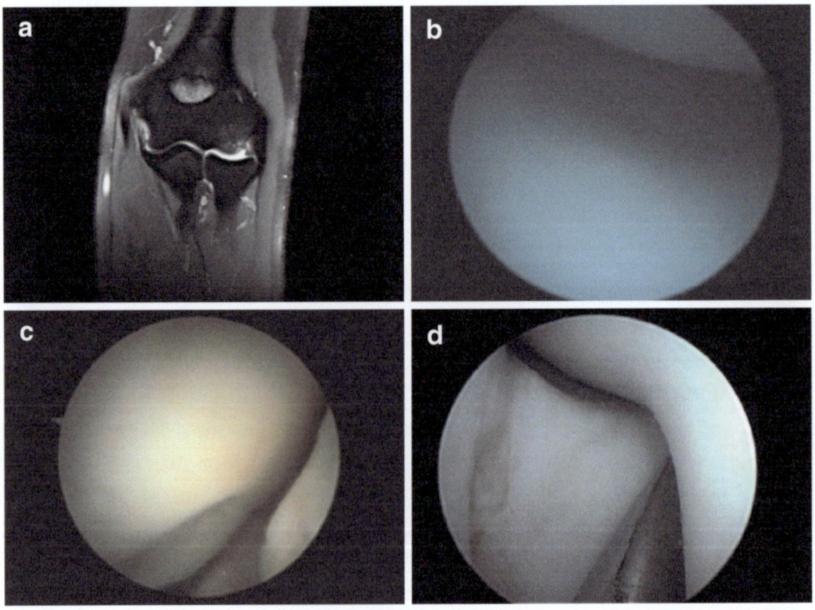

Fig. 7.2 PLRI 1°, expandability <5 mm, fixed stops. (**a**) Coronal MRI, normal; (**b**) instability test humeroradially; (**c**) instability test in the proximal radial ulnar joint (PRUJ); (**d**) instability test humeroulnar

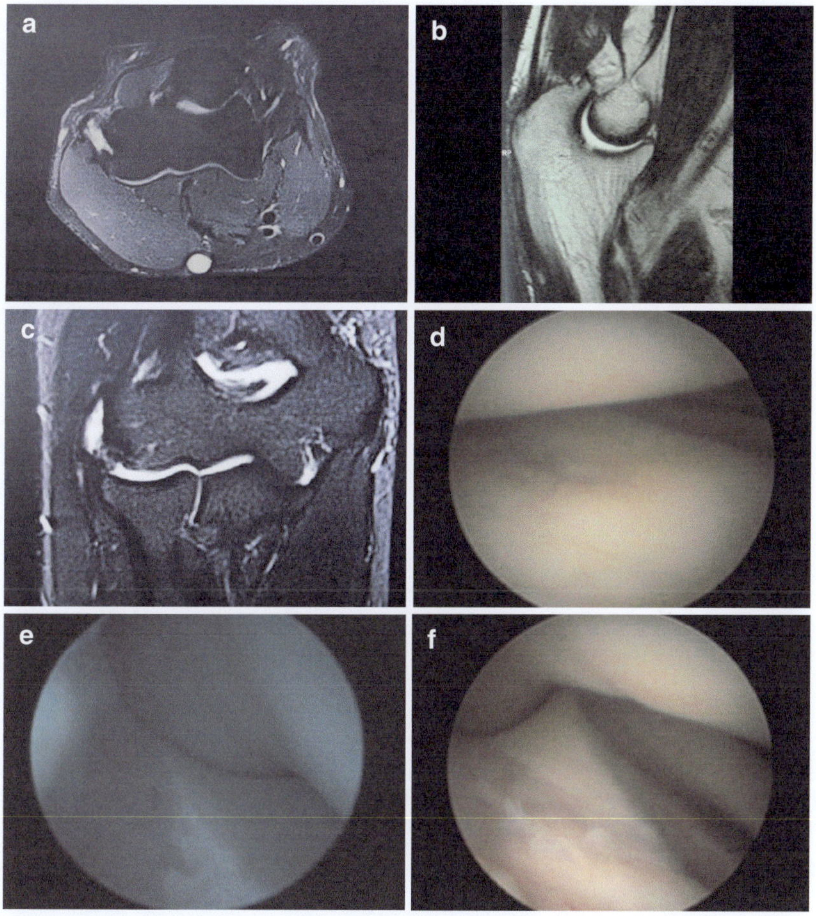

Fig. 7.3 PLRI 2°, expandability 5–10 mm, fixed stop, coronoid tip cannot be hooked. (**a**) Axial MRI gaping humeroulnar joint space; (**b**) MRI "sagittal drop sign"; (**c**) MRI coronal, extensor changes intratendinous; (**d**) instability test humeroradial with increased distance, but with stop; (**e**) humeroulnar expandability <10 mm, fixed end stop; (**f**) switching stick tip can be inserted dorsally up to the coronoid tip

can be inserted between the olecranon and trochlea. If this is possible or if this part of the joint widens spontaneously, this is positive evidence of instability (Fig. 7.4d).

The optic is now rotated along the radial olecranon while lifting the camera in the direction of the dorsolateral soft-spot portal. Here, hypertrophic synovium often appears. The dorsoradial soft-spot portal is created using the outside-in technique, and the synovium can be removed with the shaver if necessary. In case of high-grade instability, the joint space between the olecranon and humerus widens spontaneously. After establishing a good overview of the radial head and capitulum (if needed, a plica can also be resected), a switching stick or the trocar is inserted as a measuring instrument. The first check is done in the PRUG (proximal radioulnar joint); for this purpose, an attempt is made to insert the tip of the switching stick between the radial head and ulna in the PRUG. The next step is to insert the switching stick between the capitulum and the radial head. It can now be checked with the appropriate lever whether the joint can be opened in varus stress or not.

Under the same view, the assistant can perform a posterolateral rotation so that the radial head's translation can be seen under sight. Finally, the trocar is advanced between the humerus and ulna in the direction of the coronoid tip. If it is possible to "hang" on the coronoid or if the joint gap can be widened wide (>10 mm) and without a fixed point of stop, a grade 3 instability is diagnosed. If expansion is only possible up to approximately 5 mm, and if the tip of the trocar cannot be pushed over the coronoid, a grade 2 instability is diagnosed; widening that is below 5 mm varies from a stable elbow to grade 1 instability.

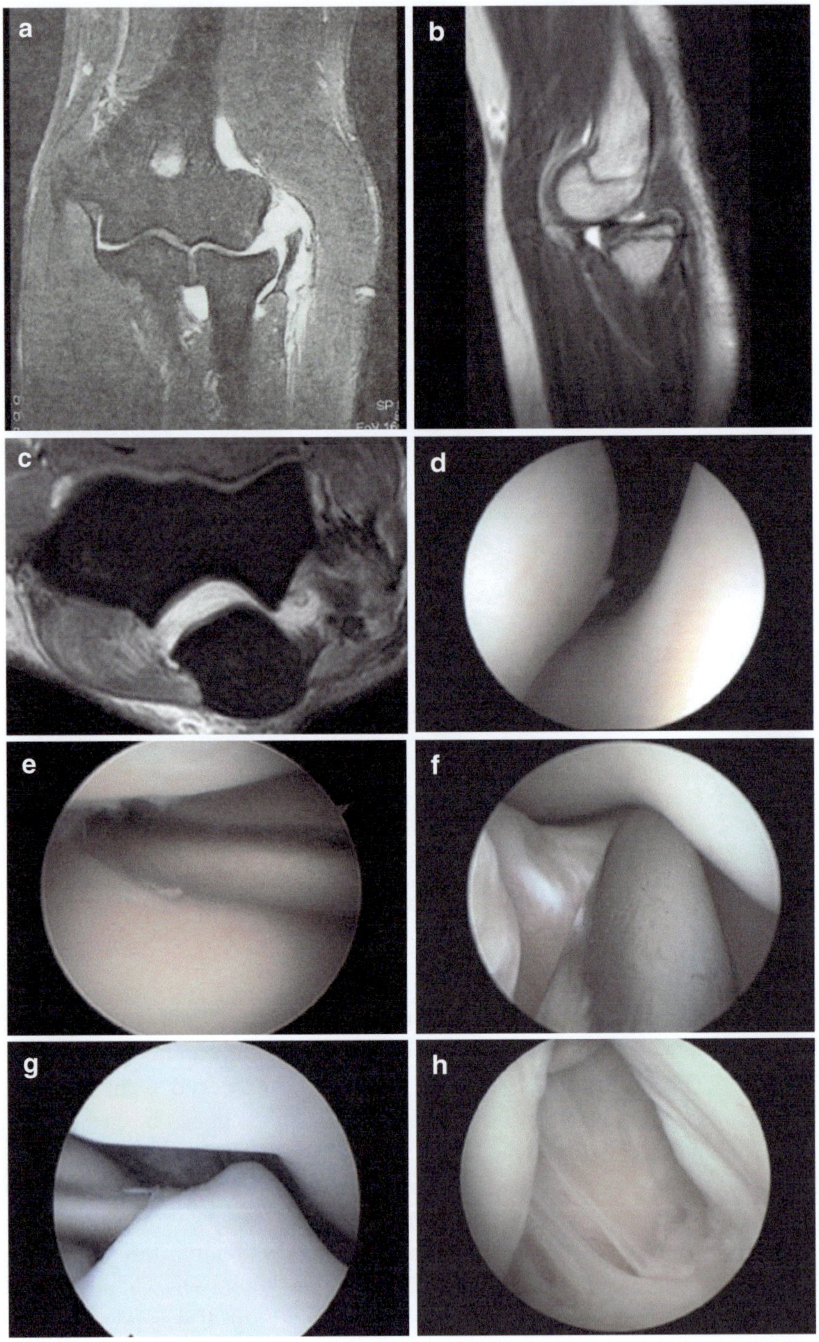

Fig. 7.4 PLRI 3°, expandability >10 mm, without a fixed stop, coronoid tip subluxable. (**a**) Coronal MRI, extensors and LUCL lesion, radial gaping; (**b**) sagittal MRI, drop sign; (**c**) Axial MRI, gaping humeroulnar gap; (**d**) Spontaneous gaping between the olecranon and humerus; (**e**) humeroradially increased expandability with positive "drive through"; (**f**) humeroulnar expandability >10 mm, no stop; (**g**) luxatable coronoid from dorsal; (**h**) extensor damage, view from intra-articular

Now, the camera portal is changed, and the flushing cannula can be used as an optic sleeve. Varus stress can be applied to the joint's medial part to rule out ulnar instability or instability combinations. The establishment of an anteromedial portal is not necessary in the context of pure instability diagnostics.

The second- and third-degree instability should be treated with a ligament reconstruction.

The arthroscopic instruments are removed, and the arm is positioned horizontally on the arm table. The dorsal portals serve as a guideline for an open approach. This occurs by including the portals in an arched manner from approximately the radial

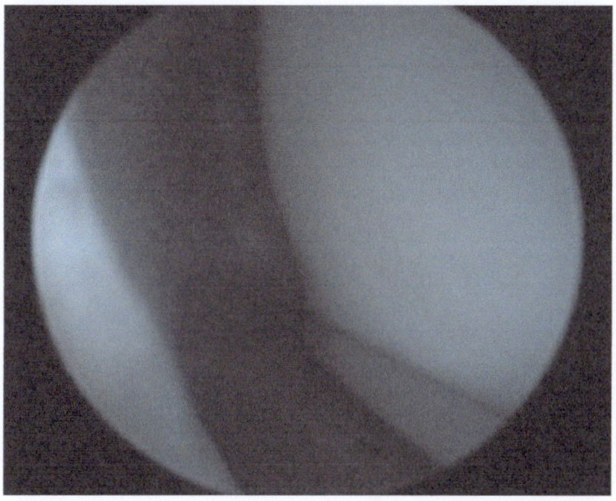

Fig. 7.5 (PRUG) Instability in the proximal radioulnar joint

head's height and directed proximally behind the epicondyle toward the triceps muscle. After incising the skin and preparing the subcutaneous tissue, the forearm fascia is exposed and split longitudinally. The fascia is then carefully mobilized anteriorly over the extensor muscle group to show the common extensor tendon. The extensors are now detached subperiosteal from the back of the epicondyle from the anconeus muscle and mobilized in the Kocher interval. The epicondyle is electrothermally denervated and refreshed.

In our approach, an approximately 7-mm-wide and 6-cm-long triceps strip is removed from the central third of the muscle, the defect is closed side to side, and the tendon is reinforced at one

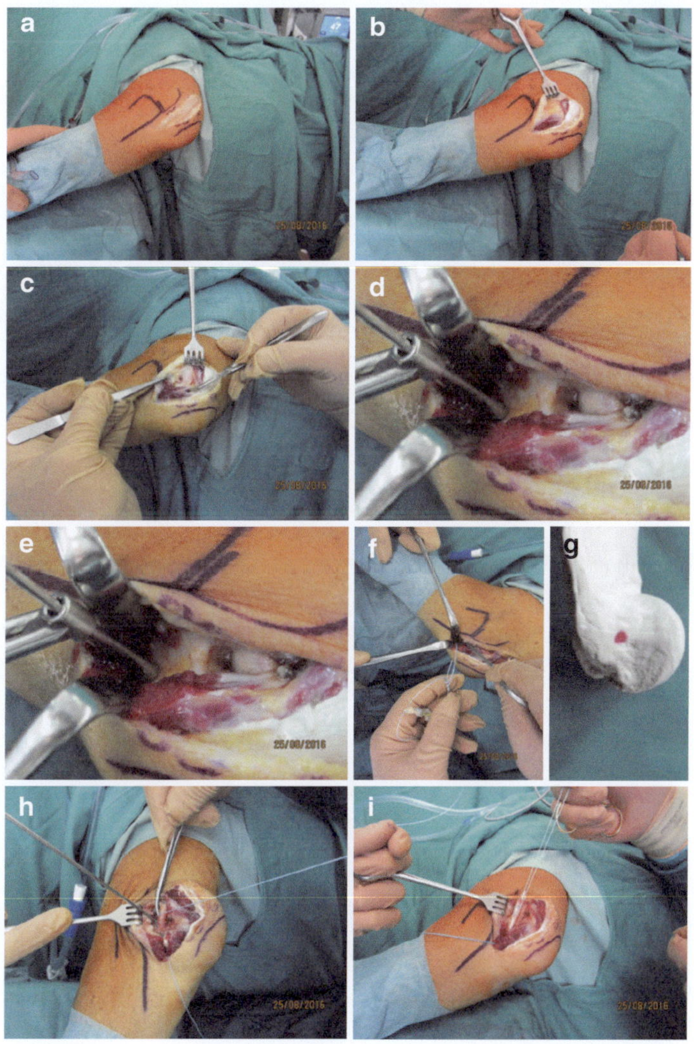

Fig. 7.6 Standard procedure for ligament repair of the lateral ulnar collateral ligament (LUCL). (**a**) incision, (**b**) splitting the forearm fascia, (**c**) access to Kocher interval with subperiosteal release from the anconeus muscle, (**d**) removal of the triceps tendon, (**e**) ulnar drilling at the level of insertion of the distal annular ligament, (**f**) insertion of the fixation button, (**g**) isometric point humeral, (**h**) isometric measurement with humeral inserted drill wire, (**i**) cutting to the required length and reinforcement, (**j**) application of the transosseous refixation threads, (**k**) LUCL fixation with 4.75 mm PEEK tenodesis screw, (**l**) Extensor fixation with Kocher interval closure and adaptation of the anconeus muscle against extensors, (**n**) closure of the forearm fascia, (**o**) post-op X-ray

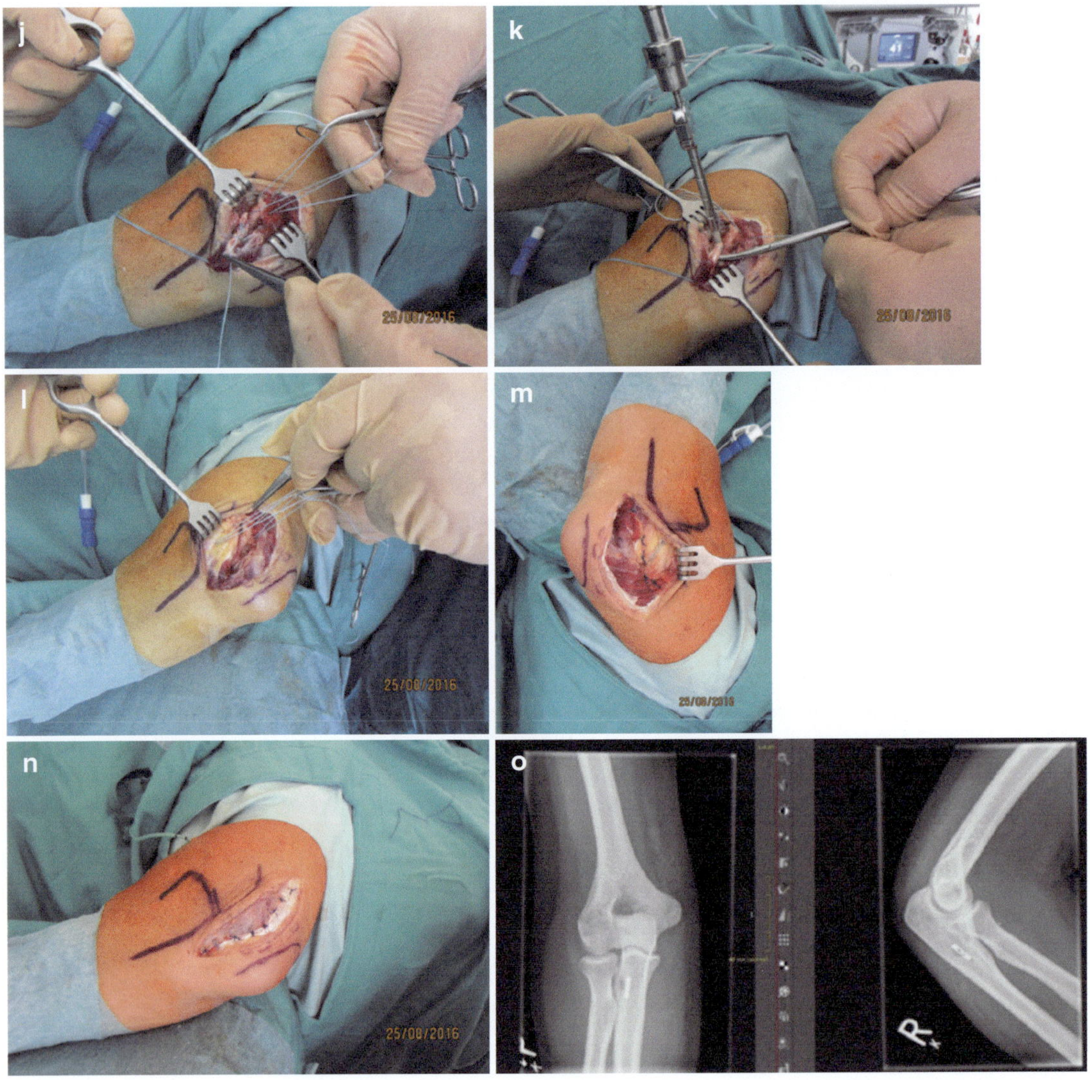

Fig. 7.6 (continued)

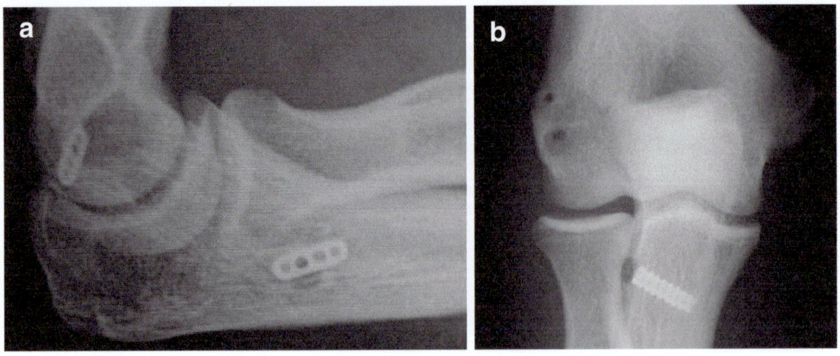

Fig. 7.7 Varieties of fixation method. (**a**) Button–Button, (**b**) Tenodesis screw–Tenodesis screw (titanium ulnar, PEEK humeral)

end with Bunnel suture with FiberWire. Palmaris or gracilis tendons can be used as revision or alternative transplants. The transplant is now fixed. The annular ligament is exposed at the Kocher interval; the first drilling is then made in the ulna at its distal attachment. The reinforcement sutures (FibreWire) passed through a biceps button (Arthrex, Naples, USA), inserted in the drilled hole, and flipped; the band is then pulled in and fixed over it. A guidewire is inserted at the insertion point of the LUCL, and the correct length is checked, and then drilling with a 5-mm drill over the drill guide wire is done. Drilling for transosseous suture is then made from the dorsal side, and an additional hole is made more proximally in the epicondyle.

The joint is reduced, the graft is adjusted to the required length, and the proximal end is reinforced with FibreWire–Bunnel sutures. After that, the graft is pulled into the hole and fixed under maximum tension with a tenodesis screw (PEEK, 4.75 mm, Arthrex). The remaining sutures are pulled out transosseously, and the detached extensors are reattached. Great care must be taken to ensure that the forearm fascia is not fixed to ensure that the layers can slide over each other. The Kocher interval is closed, and the anconeus muscle is sutured against the extensors so that the thread knots are covered. The forearm fascia is also sutured then the wound is closed in layers. Finally, a compressive bandage is applied, and an upper arm plaster splint is applied.

7.6 Follow-Up Treatment

- A perioperative interscalene pain catheter has proven its efficacy in pain management; the first 48 h, in particular, are extremely painful [10]. Postoperative radiological control should be carried out. Figure 7.7 shows the postoperative radiological images with various fixation materials.
- After 3–5 days, change to a movement-limiting orthosis (e.g., EpicoRom, Medi company, Bayreuth) as a protection tool for a total of 4 weeks. Initially, lymph drainage and passive mobilization should take place. After healing, approximately 6 weeks postoperatively, increasing strength exercises can be started. Free range of motion and good resilience can be expected approximately 3 months after the operation.

Tips and Tricks
- Arthroscopy is a diagnostic tool to classify instability.
- An isometric measurement before ligament refixation is obligatory to not cause any bending or extension inhibition or limitation.
- The joint should be freely movable after arm positioning so that the graft can be fixed with maximum tension.
- If the band was harvested too short, stable fixation via a tenodesis screw is risky. In this case, additional securing is required; this can be achieved with reinforcement sutures with button augmentation.
- If the removed graft is too long, it will not be possible to build up enough tension.
- If the diameter of the transplant is too large, it will not be possible to pull it inadequately, or the tenodesis screw may not grip adequately.

References

1. Josefsson PO, Nilsson BE. Incidence of elbow dislocation. Acta Orthop Scand. 1986;57(6):537–8.
2. Geyer M, Schoch C, Harnoss T. Therapiemöglichkeiten der chronischen ligamentären Ellbogeninstabilität. Arthroskopie. 2013;26(3):197–206.
3. O'Driscoll SW, Bell DF, Morrey BF. Posterolateral rotatory instability of the elbow. J Bone Joint Surg Am. 1991;73(3):440–6.
4. Camp CL, O'Driscoll SW, Wempe MK, Smith J. The sonographic posterolateral rotatory stress test for elbow instability: a cadaveric validation study. PM R. 2017;9(3):275–82.
5. Eygendaal D, Valstar ER, Söjbjerg JO, Rozing PM. Biomechanical evaluation of the elbow using roentgen stereophotogrammetric analysis. Clin Orthop Relat Res. 2002;396:100–5.
6. O'Brien MJ, Savoie FH 3rd. Arthroscopic and open management of posterolateral rotatory instability of the elbow. Sports Med Arthrosc Rev. 2014;22(3):194–200.
7. VanRiet RP. Arthroscopic LUCL augmentation. Lecture International Advanced Course on Elbow Surgery (IAECS) Madrid; 2015.

8. O'Driscoll SW, Morrey BF, Korinek S, An KN. Elbow subluxation dislocation: a spectrum of instability. Clin Orthop Relat Res. 1992;280:186–97.
9. Cain EL Jr, Dugas JR, Wolf RS, Andrews JR. Elbow injuries in throwing athletes: a current concepts review. Am J Sports Med. 2003;31(4):621–35.
10. Schoch C. Learning curve in Ellbogen-Arthroskopie und LUCLBandplastik – eine persönliche Studie. Lecture Gesellschaft für Arthroskopie und Gelenk chirurgie (AGA), Jahreskongress Innsbruck; 2014.

Arthroscopic Treatment for Elbow Osteoarthritis

8

K. Wegmann, M. Hackl, and L. P. Müller

Contents

8.1 Pathology

Elbow osteoarthritis can be a painful disease that significantly restricts the functionality and thus the quality of life of the entire affected limb. Even if it is assumed that the elbow is exposed to less loads than the knee or hip joint, primary osteoarthritic changes can occur. However, secondary posttraumatic arthritis of the elbow is much more common. In addition to posttraumatic arthritis, secondary osteoarthritis of the elbow can also develop due to infectious, rheumatic, and osteonecrotic changes. The diagnosis and arthroscopic therapy of primary and posttraumatic osteoarthritis are presented below.

Primary elbow osteoarthritis is rare and represents only 2–3% of osteoarthritis changes in the elbow. It usually manifests itself initially in the ulnohumeral joint in patients who are subjected to physical stress through sport or work, but also through mobility associated with a wheelchair or crutches. Typically, it is found in the dominant extremity of men aged 40–50 years. The ulnohumeral joint shows a high degree of osseous congruence. In maximum extension and flexion, the bony structures can come to an abrupt stop. Primary osteoarthritis often shows itself initially through osteophyte formation at the tip of the olecranon or the tip of the coronoid process. Examples of this are combat sports athletes who are exposed to corresponding hyperextension

K. Wegmann (✉)
OCM (Orthopädische Chirurgie München) Clinic, München, Germany
e-mail: kilian.wegmann@ocm-muenchen.de

M. Hackl · L. P. Müller
Department of Orthopedic and Trauma Surgery, University Hospital Cologne, Cologne, Germany
e-mail: michael.hackl@uk-koeln.de; lars.mueller@uk-koeln.de

A. B. Imhoff, A. Lenich (eds.), *Elbow Arthroscopy and Minimal Invasive Surgery*,
https://doi.org/10.1007/978-3-031-75611-5_8

through forced extension when striking. On the other hand, excessive flexion is found, for example, in weight lifters or goalkeepers. Another example is the builder or mechanic who often has to lift and support heavy loads overhead.

As the disease progresses, the ulnohumeral joint remains apart from the osteophytes of the olecranon and the coronoid. Then, the osteoarthritis extends to the radial part of the joint, an isolated primary osteoarthritis of the radiohumeral joint being less common, and it usually occurs at the head of the radius below a hypertrophic posterolateral plica. In advanced osteoarthritis, both the radial and ulnar compartments are affected.

There are multiple explanations for the specific genesis of primary osteoarthritis, as the etiology has not yet been fully understood in detail. Due to the mechanical loading and overloading of the cartilage, a complex cascade between inflammatory mediators and nociceptive stimulation is presumably triggered, which leads to progressive destruction of the joint surfaces and pain [1].

In secondary posttraumatic osteoarthritis, which is much more common than the primary form, there is usually traumatic cartilage damage or an incongruence of the joint surfaces. The articular cartilage is weakened, causing osteoarthritis to develop. Different elbow fractures vary in the risk of secondary osteoarthritis. Guitton et al. retrospectively analyzed 139 patients after elbow trauma to quantify the various risks [2]. They identified the fracture type as an independent risk factor for the development of posttraumatic elbow osteoarthritis. In particular, fractures of the distal humerus and dislocation fractures showed a high probability of developing osteoarthritis. Up to 80% of patients with a distal humerus fracture seem to suffer from secondary osteoarthritis [3].

Male patients are affected significantly and more frequently by both primary and secondary elbow osteoarthritis. Primary osteoarthritis affects the dominant extremity first in more than 80% of cases, and bilateral involvement is found in about 60% of the cases. The complaints of those patients usually occur in the primarily affected regions. The osteophytes of the olecranon and the coronoid tip can lead to pain and crepitus sensation in extension or flexion. Radiohumeral osteoarthritis is typically painful when the radial joint is mechanically loaded and during rotation. However, the clinical manifestation of elbow osteoarthritis is not always complementary to the imaging findings of joint damage. Depending on the native radiological images, primary osteoarthritis (according to Hastings and Rettig) and posttraumatic osteoarthritis (according to Broberg and Morrey) were divided into three degrees of severity [4].

However, severe forms of osteoarthritis with pronounced narrowing of the joint space and osteophyte formation can be presented with only moderate clinical symptoms. Loose joint bodies can lead to entrapment and stabbing pain. If the affected person experiences pain over the entire range of motion and not only with terminal flexion or extension, this can also indicate advanced destruction of the central part of the joint surface of the radiohumeral or ulnohumeral joints. A disturbed movement pattern with regard to the axis of rotation can be related to elbow osteoarthritis. Miyake et al. studied the movement pattern of the elbow in patients with primary osteoarthritis using CT data [5]. It was found that patients with radiohumeral osteoarthritis have a bigger valgus angle during flexion than healthy elbows. This underlines the relevance of the degenerative pathology of osteoarthritis, which has a self-reinforcing character due to the malposition and the associated peak loads.

Patients with elbow osteoarthritis often have accompanying symptoms like affection of the ulnar nerve [6]. In a healthy elbow, it has been shown that flexion increases the pressure in the ulnar groove by narrowing it by around 45% [7]. In 2014, Kawanishi and colleagues reported a relationship between the structure of the distal, medial humerus osteophytes and the occurrence of ulnar symptoms [8]. Direct mechanical irritation of the nerve by osteophytes seems to be the cause. The ulnar nerve and the supplied areas must be clinically examined.

8.2 Indication

Treatment of elbow osteoarthritis ranges from conservative treatment with physiotherapy, the use of splints, and “Continuous Passive Motion” (CPM) to joint replacement. If a relevant joint stiffness persists for 6 months despite conservative treatment, surgical therapy is then indicated. The prosthetic replacement provides good pain reduction and increased mobility but comes at the expense of costs, durability, and upcoming replacement operations. Surgical Interventions aimed to debride the joint and therefore delay the need for replacement operations. However, the indication for surgery must be tailored to the patient. Removal of osteophytes can destabilize the joint and further accelerate the degenerative process that was initiated as a result of chronic instability.

Open procedures for debridement of the elbow in osteoarthritis have been described several times; clinical studies have reported successful results with pain reduction and improved mobility [9–12]. Arthroscopic therapy for elbow osteoarthritis has developed and established itself over the past few years [13–17]. In 2000, Cohen and his colleagues compared the outcome of 44 patients, of whom 18 had undergone open and 26 had undergone arthroscopic debridement of the elbow [18]. The authors found a better reduction in the flexion deficit with the open approach, and there were no other significant differences between the two methods. In a prospective study on arthroscopic arthrolysis, Cefo and Eygendaal showed an improvement in the range of motion from 99° to 125°, with a low rate of complications [19].

After arthroscopic joint debridement, however, there is a risk of iatrogenic nerve damage. A large number of case reports and case series exist in the literature [20–27], which describe the corresponding damage to single or even several peripheral nerves around the elbow. Precise knowledge of the anatomy and a standardized surgical procedure are essential to optimize the safety of the procedure. In general, it must be taken in mind that posttraumatic arthrosis or previously operated joints, due to the scarring, entail a significantly higher risk of iatrogenic nerve damage and are therefore only conditionally accessible to arthroscopic therapy or only with appropriate experience. As with all other arthroscopic interventions, it is essential to master complementary open procedures to allow for conversion in the case of difficulties that may occur during the arthroscopy.

8.3 Operating Principle/Instruments

On one hand, the operation aims to remove the conflicting osteophytes [28]. The relevant osteophytes are usually found at the mechanically exposed, prominent points such as the tip of the olecranon and the coronoid, as well as on the corresponding areas of the olecranon and coronoid fossa. In addition, osteophytes which are found in the radial fossa are caused by repetitive strokes or loads on the radial head. In addition, the arthritic elbow often has osteophytes at the radial and ulnar olecranon edges. Like olecranon tip osteophytes, these can be an obstacle to extension. All osteophytes can be resected with a shaver or arthroscopic forceps and also with a chisel. It should be noted, however, that reaching the osteophytes with surgical instruments can be extremely demanding. In particular, debridement in the ulnar recess is complex, and it is linked to immediate iatrogenic damage to the ulnar nerve. Free joint loose bodies should be removed, as they can cause pinching and blocking of the joint with shooting pain. Cartilage therapy for degenerative damage is limited.

Smoothing out of the protruded cartilage or fraying of cartilage can also help to reduce the pain. Microfracture as a therapy for cartilage lesions has been used for many years. There is evidence of its effectiveness, particularly in the knee joint, but it has a limited duration of pain reduction [29, 30]. Another benefit of arthroscopic debridement is the treatment of the joint stiffness. Partially, through the removal of the osteophytes, which are not only pain generators, but also by acting as mechanical obstacles to joint movement. Resection of the joint capsule ventrally and dorsally can also improve mobility.

Neurolysis of the ulnar nerve should be performed openly or endoscopically before the procedure if symptoms arise. It is recommended to perform this before the arthroscopy, as the localization of the nerve facilitates debridement in the medial recess. Furthermore, neurolysis is easier to perform before the arthroscopic fluid swells the soft tissues.

The standard set of instruments for arthroscopic debridement should include the following:

- Vacuum mattress, alternatively sacrum, and symphysis pubis support.
- Armrest.
- Towels, if necessary, a warming blanket, plexus pillows.
- Tourniquet (the use of a tourniquet is possible, but not absolutely necessary needed).
- Sterile skin markers.
- Puncture cannula (e.g., 20 G), bone pliers.
- Scalpel no. 11.
- Dissecting scissors.
- Inflow cannula.
- Trocar sleeve with a blunt trocar.
- Arthroscopy tower with camera and video processor, documents station unit, pump, light source, optic.
- Shaver unit with 3.5-mm soft tissue shaver and 4.0-mm bone cutter.
- Diathermy.
- Fine chisels (0.6–2.0 cm wide), hammer.
- Arthroscopic forceps (grasping forceps, arthroscopic scissors, punches, e.g., 45° right/left), rongeur (from spine surgery instrument set).
- Elevator, e.g., 4 mm and 8 mm.
- K-wires 1.6–2.0.
- Curved awl in 30°, 40°, 60°.
- 3/0 nonabsorbable suture.
- If necessary, add extensions/flexions splints cast/slab, alternatively brace.

8.4 Preparation for Surgery

In addition to the usual medical history, the following points must be clarified preoperatively:

- Skin condition in the area to be operated.
- Preexisting incisions/scars.
- Bony deformities, posttraumatic pathological joint incongruence, pseudarthroses, bony defects (CT!).
- *Status of the ulnar nerve*: here, it is inevitable to know whether previous operations have been performed or even a transposition of the ulnar nerve has been carried out. If the location of the nerve after previous operations is questionable, an exploration with localization should be considered (reference in the surgical clarification should be documented). External surgical reports can also be incorrect in connection with the position of the ulnar nerve and can mislead the revising surgeon.
- Joint stability?
- Existing implants/osteosynthesis material (manufacturer, status, location).
- Heterotopic ossifications.

The intervention takes place in the lateral decubitus position. The lateral position is usually not tolerated for a long time by the awake patient, which is why the procedure is performed under general anesthesia. Additional plexus anesthesia is advisable, especially for interventions that require rapid and intensive postoperative physiotherapy, for example, stiffness. The patient is placed in a vacuum mattress on the healthy side. The arm to be operated on is placed in an arm holder (e.g., Ontario arm holder); no further fixation is required to freely move the operated extremity intraoperatively. Alternatively, the patient can be stabilized without a vacuum mattress with the aid of the sacrum and symphysis pubis supports. Furthermore, it is important to position the healthy extremities relaxed and without pressure, the use of a plexus cushion under healthy lying is desirable. Perioperative antibiotics should be administered before a tourniquet is applied.

8.5 Surgical Technique

After marking the anatomical landmarks, the joint is filled with sterile saline solution (20–30 mL).

Caution: In case of degenerative changes, stiffness, and so on, the volume can be significantly reduced. In a healthy joint, the fluid is distributed in the dorsal or ventral compartment throughout the joint after injection. In the arthritic joint with osteophytes and stiffness, the communication between the spaces may be disturbed. The irrigation cannula is placed through the proximal anterolateral portal. If an optimal rinsing effect is required in front of the camera, the fluid can also be supplied via the trocar.

We begin the arthroscopy dorsally through the high posterolateral portal and the transtricipital portal. The portals can be changed during the procedure to optimize the view or the working angle of the instruments. It is also possible to create auxiliary portals under strict observation of the neurovascular structures. Dorsally, synovitis and fibrotic adhesions are usually found in the arthritis elbow. To visualize the osteophytes and free joint loose bodies, these soft tissue adhesions should be resected. We start with the camera in the high posterolateral portal and the shaver through the transtricipital portal. With the shaver opening turned laterally, the adhesions are resected. Beginning at the radial border of the fossa, continue cranially and then medially (Figs. 8.1, 8.2, and 8.3). Whenever the boundary is shown, work is carried out from there toward the center of the fossa floor. It is imperative to pay the greatest possible attention to protect the ulnar nerve. The nerve must be expected in the ulnar recess immediately medial to the joint capsule. After the soft tissues have been resected, exposed osteophytes or free loose bodies should be resected or removed (Figs. 8.4 and 8.5). If there are osteophytes in the olecranon, they are removed with a burr or chisel (Figs. 8.6, 8.7, and 8.8). At the medial edge of the olecranon, however, extreme caution must be taken in order not to endanger the ulnar nerve. If difficulties arise here, it is advisable to expose the ulnar nerve or to proceed openly. These two extensions of the operation must be noted and documented in the patient's clarification, and the patient must have been informed and agreed preoperatively.

After finishing the dorsal debridement, the camera is transferred into the radiohumeral joint. After the camera has been brought into the so-called triangle between the radial head, the olecranon, and the capitulum, a deep posterolateral portal is created in the soft spot. The shaver or electrocautery can now be introduced.

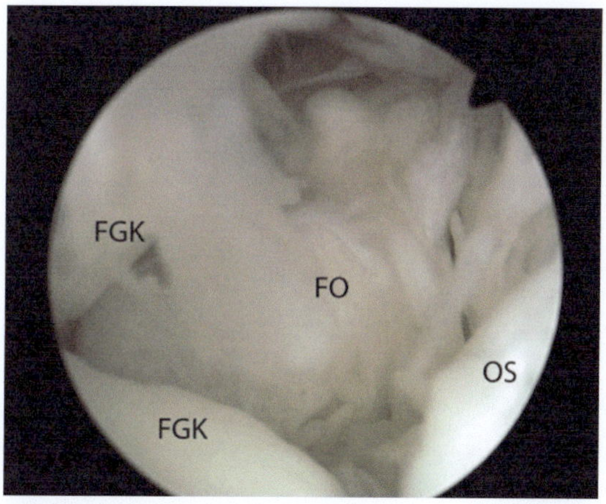

Fig. 8.1 Adhesions in the fossa (FO) with free joint loose bodies (FGK) and osteophytes (OS)

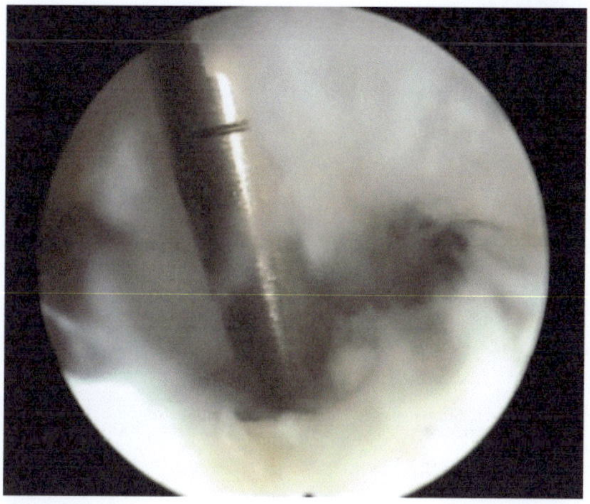

Fig. 8.2 Resection of the adhesions and synovitis

It is possible to change the portals between the camera and the working instruments or to create auxiliary portals if necessary. The synovitis and fibrotic scarring are also debrided here. In advanced osteoarthritis, especially secondary osteoarthritis and previous osteosynthesis of the radial head, severe scarring could be found here (Fig. 8.9). Free loose bodies are freed from soft tissue and removed (Fig. 8.10). If there is localized arthritis, drilling of the defect at the head of the radius or at the capitulum with opening of the subchondral medullary canal (microfracture) can enable the formation of fibrocartilage. For this

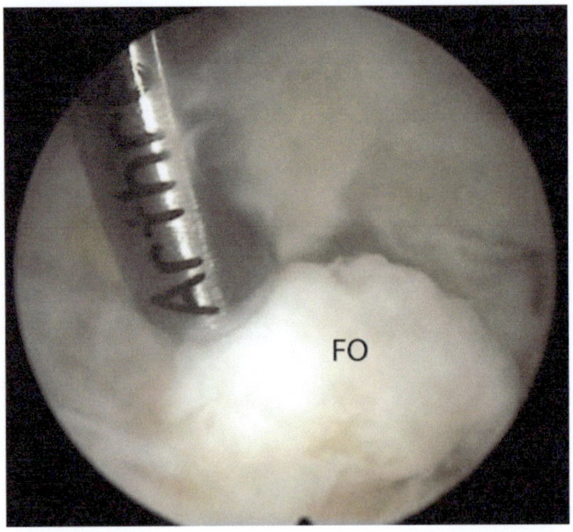

Fig. 8.3 The solid osteophyte (FO) can be isolated on the fossa floor

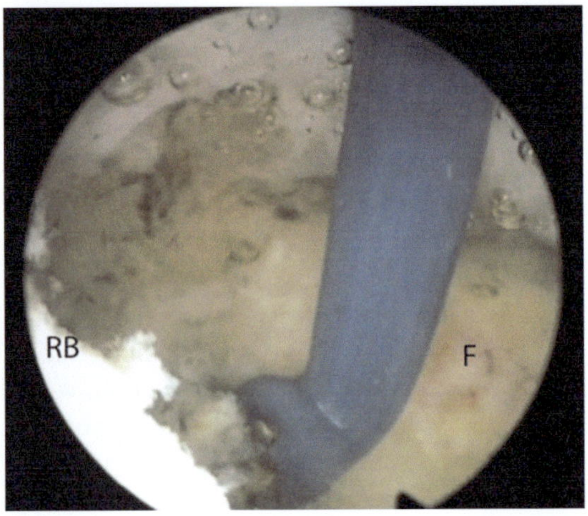

Fig. 8.5 The fossa floor is then freed of any remaining soft tissue using electrocautery. *F* fossa, *RB* radial border of the fossa

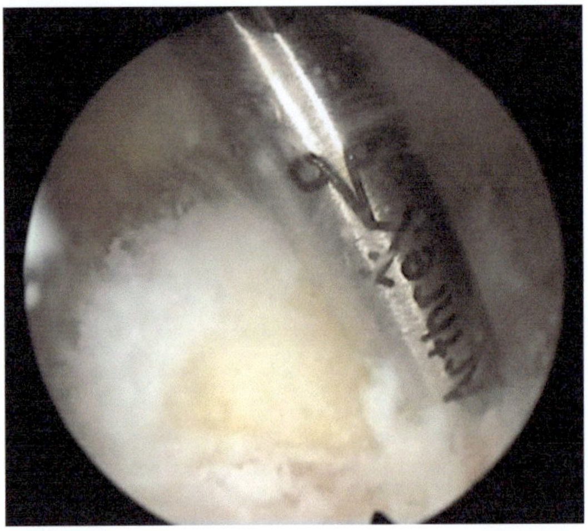

Fig. 8.4 The osteophyte is resected with the bone bur

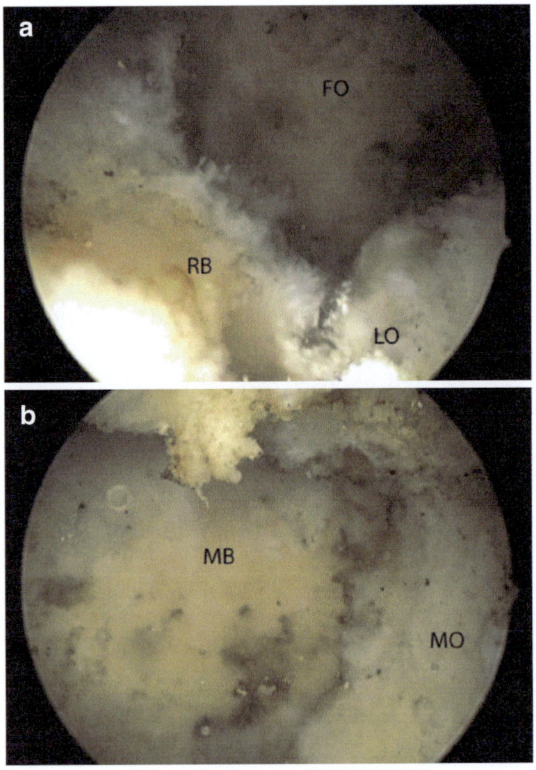

Fig. 8.6 (**a**) An osteophyte of the lateral olecranon (LO) protrudes over the radial boundary (RB) of the olecranon fossa (FO). (**b**) Medially shows a complementary picture. *MB* medial edge of the fossa, *MO* medial olecranon

purpose, small openings (e.g., K-wire 1.6 mm or curved awl) are drilled with a distance of 3–4 mm between them in the area of the defect until droplets of cancellous fatty tissue emerge.

If the arthroscopic fluid is turned off, blood leakage can be observed from the opening of the microfracture. In the case of advanced degeneration of the radial head with clinical evidence of radial elbow pain, resection of the radial head is a possible treatment option [31]. The indication must be taken strictly because

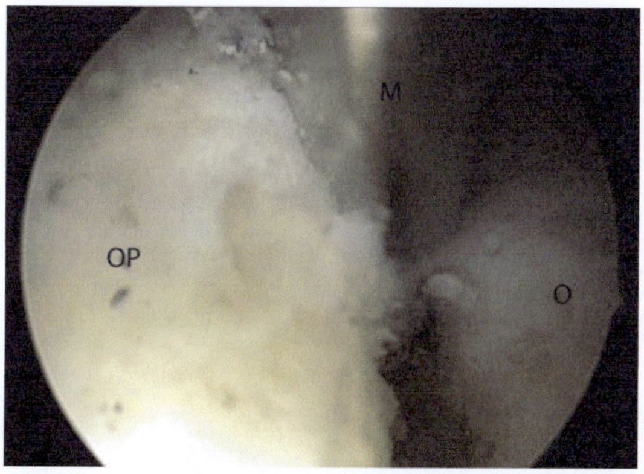

Fig. 8.7 The osteophyte (OP) is separated from the medial olecranon (O) with the chisel (M)

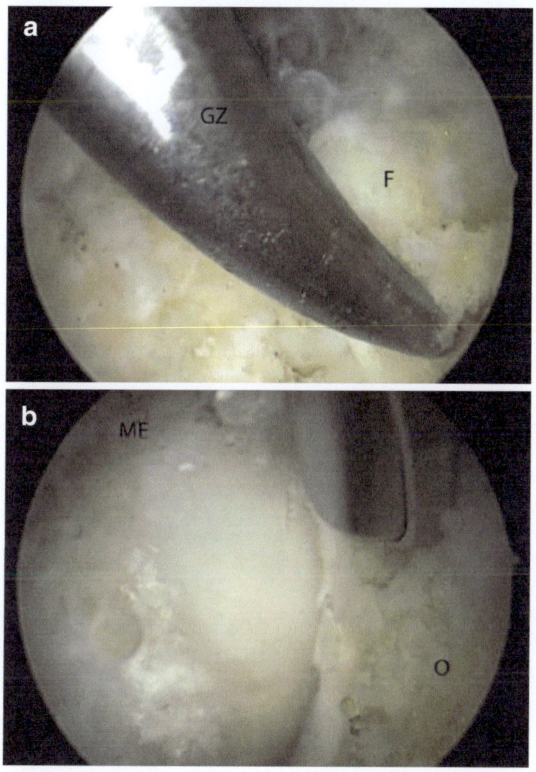

Fig. 8.8 (**a**) After retrieving the fragment (F) with the grasping forceps (GZ) and after smoothing with the shaver, the medial epicondyle (ME) and the trochlea are freed (with the elbow flexed) (**b**)

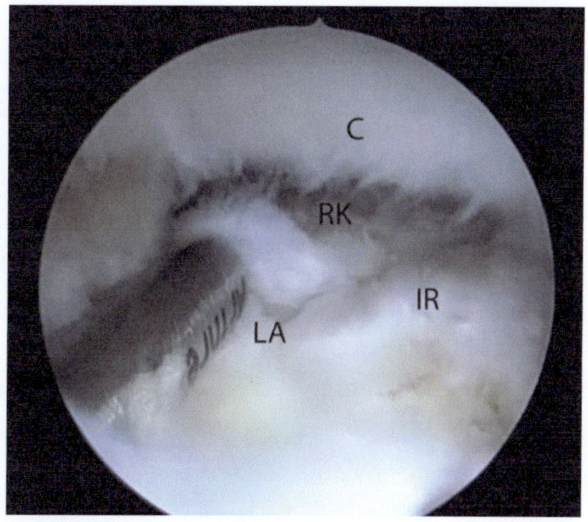

Fig. 8.9 View from the high posterolateral portal of the radial head (RK), the capitulum (C), the radial notch (IR), and the posterior portion of the annular ligament (LA) in a left elbow. Only after soft tissue debridement with the shaver is it possible to see clearly the degenerated bony structures

accelerated ulnohumeral degeneration and valgus compensation have been observed after the radius head resection. Resection of the radial head is possible arthroscopically and is associated with reduced morbidity and a comparable surgery time. For the OP technique, see Figs. 8.11, 8.12, and 8.13.

In our own technique, a drainage is inserted after the operative procedure when a wide bone surface has been opened and the risk of a hematoma formation is increased. After the portals have been sutured (e.g., with a 3/0 simple suture), a sterile wound dressing and an elastocompressive wrapping are applied. If there was a stiffness preoperatively, an extending or flexing orthosis is put on.

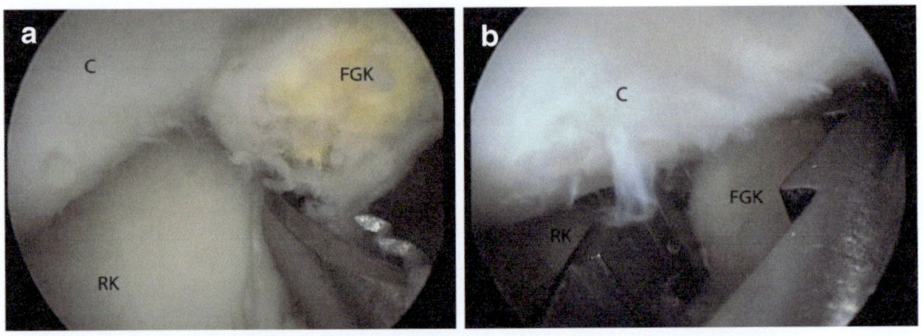

Fig. 8.10 (**a**) A free joint loose body (FGK) is clamped between the capitulum (C), olecranon (covered by the FGK), and radial head (RK). (**b**) This is retrieved with the grasping forceps

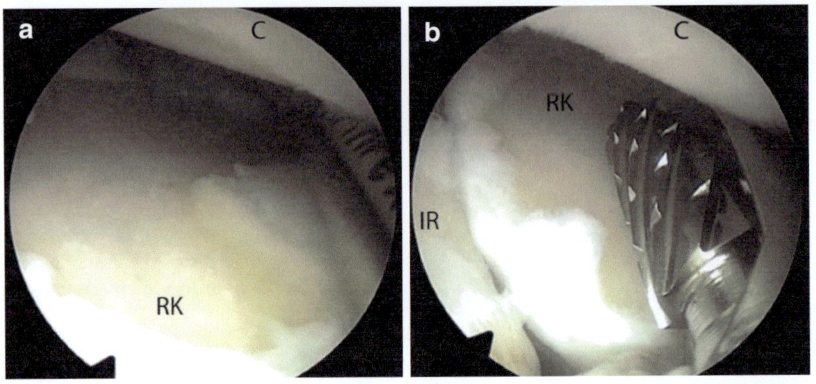

Fig. 8.11 (**a**) Before the resection, arthritic degeneration of the radial head (RK) and of the humeral capitulum (C). (**b**) We begin the resection at the ulnar edge of the radial head (RK) in a neutral position. The ulna borders the radial notch (IR). In our own approach, we prefer to use an oval milling cutter, in contrast to a round milling cutter, as the oval milling cutter allows milling a larger area and simultaneously accelerate the procedure

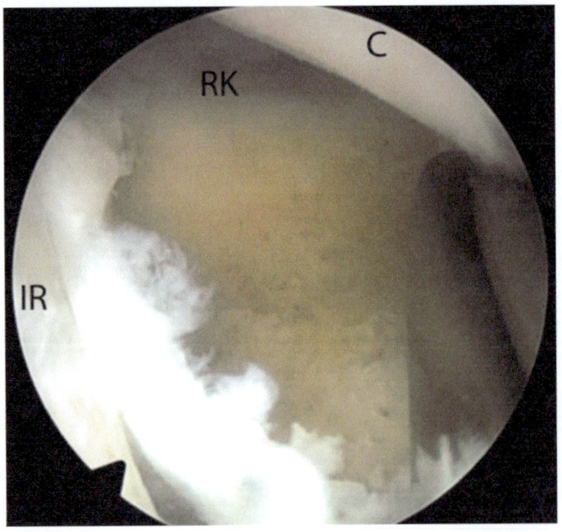

Fig. 8.12 The radial head is resected in horizontal movements. By rotating the forearm, the anterior areas can be brought into the working area of the shaver. The cartilaginous wall of the neck, which is often at the edge of the neck and cannot be easily reached with the shaver, is removed with punches or grasping forceps. *C* capitulum, *IR* radial notch, *RK* radius head

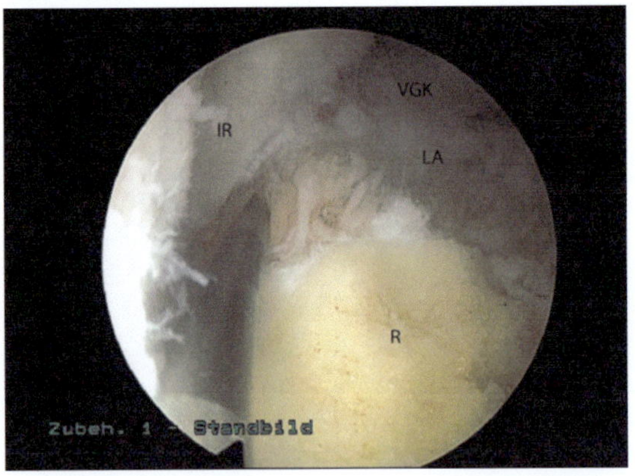

Fig. 8.13 The lower edge of the radial notch (IR) is palpated with the hook. In our own technique, the resection is carried up just above this height. Finally, rinsing should be carried out in order to remove the fragments and debris. *IR* radial notch, *R* radius, *LA* annular ligament, *VGK* ventral joint compartment

8.6 Postoperative Measures

If there is a history of heterotopic ossification, we recommend a prophylaxis with indomethacin. Cooling should take place during the first 48 h after the procedure. Elevation and lymphatic drainage begin immediately after the operation. Pain therapy is based on the WHO-level scheme. The support of pain therapy with a preoperative plexus block (e.g., with ropivacaine) is recommended.

If a stiff elbow has been treated, the corresponding physiotherapy exercise is started immediately. If extensive bone has been resected and destabilization is possible, the extremity is prevented from loads for 12 weeks.

Tips and Tricks

- When establishing the indication, the patient's expectations must be carefully evaluated. Debridement is a symptomatic treatment option, but not a treatment of the cause.
- The tourniquet leads to reduced bleeding during the procedure, which allows a better overview, especially if the cancellous bone is opened during debridement. However, their use is not absolutely necessary.
- When working with high-frequency devices, especially when resecting the radial head, a large amount of debris occurs in a short time, which can block the view. It is necessary to maintain the view with alternating suction and rinsing maneuvers.
- When grasping small free joint bodies, it can be helpful to stop the flow of fluid to stop the fragments from moving.
- The pump pressure should always be kept as low as possible to minimize swelling of the soft tissues.

References

1. Dimitroulas T, Duarte RV, Behura A, Kitas GD, Raphael JH. Neuropathic pain in osteoarthritis: a review of pathophysiological mechanisms and implications for treatment. Semin Arthritis Rheum. 2014;44(2):145–54. https://doi.org/10.1016/j.semarthrit.2014.05.011.
2. Guitton TG, Zurakowski D, van Dijk NC, Ring D. Incidence and risk factors for the development of radiographic arthrosis after traumatic elbow injuries. J Hand Surg Am. 2010;35(12):1976–80. https://doi.org/10.1016/j.jhsa.2010.08.010.
3. Doornberg JN, van Duijn PJ, Linzel D, et al. Surgical treatment of intra-articular fractures of the distal part of the humerus. Functional outcome after twelve to thirty years. J Bone Joint Surg Am. 2007;89(7):1524–32. https://doi.org/10.2106/JBJS.F.00369.
4. Amini MH, Sykes JB, Olson ST, et al. Reliability testing of two classification systems for osteoarthritis and post-traumatic arthritis of the elbow. J Shoulder Elb Surg. 2015;24(3):353–7. https://doi.org/10.1016/j.jse.2014.10.015.
5. Miyake J, Shimada K, Moritomo H, Kataoka T, Murase T, Sugamoto K. Kinematic changes in elbow osteoarthritis: in vivo and 3-dimensional analysis using computed tomographic data. J Hand Surg Am. 2013;38(5):957–64. https://doi.org/10.1016/j.jhsa.2013.02.006.
6. Kato H, Hirayama T, Minami A, Iwasaki N, Hirachi K. Cubital tunnel syndrome associated with medial elbow Ganglia and osteoarthritis of the elbow. J Bone Joint Surg Am. 2002;84-A(8):1413–9.
7. Gelberman RH, Yamaguchi K, Hollstien SB, et al. Changes in interstitial pressure and cross-sectional area of the cubital tunnel and of the ulnar nerve with flexion of the elbow. An experimental study in human cadavera. J Bone Joint Surg Am. 1998;80(4):492–501.
8. Kawanishi Y, Miyake J, Omori S, Murase T, Shimada K. The association between cubital tunnel morphology and ulnar neuropathy in patients with elbow osteoarthritis. J Shoulder Elb Surg. 2014;23(7):938–45. https://doi.org/10.1016/j.jse.2014.01.047.
9. Oka Y, Ohta K, Saitoh I. Debridement arthroplasty for osteoarthritis of the elbow. Clin Orthop Relat Res. 1998;351:127–34.
10. Tsuge K, Mizuseki T. Debridement arthroplasty for advanced primary osteoarthritis of the elbow. Results of a new technique used for 29 elbows. J Bone Joint Surg Br. 1994;76(4):641–6.
11. Vingerhoeds B, Degreef I, De Smet L. Debridement arthroplasty for osteoarthritis of the elbow (outer-bridge-Kashiwagi procedure). Acta Orthop Belg. 2004;70(4):306–10.
12. Wada T, Isogai S, Ishii S, Yamashita T. Debridement arthroplasty for primary osteoarthritis of the elbow. J Bone Joint Surg Am. 2004;86-A(2):233–41.
13. Liu YJ, Wang JL, Li HF, Qi W, Wang N. Efficacies of arthroscopic debridement and olecranon fossa plasty in the treatment of osteoarthritis and posterior elbow impingement. Zhonghua Yi Xue Za Zhi. 2012;92(27):1913–5.
14. MacLean SB, Oni T, Crawford LA, Deshmukh SC. Medium-term results of arthroscopic debridement and capsulectomy for the treatment of elbow

osteoarthritis. J Shoulder Elb Surg. 2013;22(5):653–7. https://doi.org/10.1016/j.jse.2013.01.030.
15. O'Driscoll SW. Arthroscopic treatment for osteoarthritis of the elbow. Orthop Clin North Am. 1995;26(4):691–706.
16. Ogilvie-Harris DJ, Gordon R, MacKay M. Arthroscopic treatment for posterior impingement in degenerative arthritis of the elbow. Arthroscopy. 1995;11(4):437–43.
17. Redden JF, Stanley D. Arthroscopic fenestration of the olecranon fossa in the treatment of osteoarthritis of the elbow. Arthroscopy. 1993;9(1):14–6.
18. Cohen AP, Redden JF, Stanley D. Treatment of osteoarthritis of the elbow: a comparison of open and arthroscopic debridement. Arthroscopy. 2000;16(7):701–6.
19. Cefo I, Eygendaal D. Arthroscopic arthrolysis for posttraumatic elbow stiffness. J Shoulder Elb Surg. 2011;20(3):434–9. https://doi.org/10.1016/j.jse.2010.11.018.
20. Dumonski ML, Arciero RA, Mazzocca AD. Ulnar nerve palsy after elbow arthroscopy. Arthroscopy. 2006;22(5):577.e1–3. https://doi.org/10.1016/j.arthro.2005.12.049.
21. Gupta A, Sunil Tm T. Complete division of the posterior interosseous nerve after elbow arthroscopy: a case report. J Shoulder Elb Surg. 2004;13(5):566–7. https://doi.org/10.1016/S1058274604000503.
22. Haapaniemi T, Berggren M, Adolfsson L. Complete transection of the median and radial nerves during arthroscopic release of post-traumatic elbow contracture. Arthroscopy. 1999;15(7):784–7.
23. Hahn M, Grossman JA. Ulnar nerve laceration as a result of elbow arthroscopy. J Hand Surg Br. 1998;23(1):109.
24. Kelly EW, Morrey BF, O'Driscoll SW. Complications of elbow arthroscopy. J Bone Joint Surg Am. 2001;83-A(1):25–34.
25. Nelson GN, Wu T, Galatz LM, Yamaguchi K, Keener JD. Elbow arthroscopy: early complications and associated risk factors. J Shoulder Elb Surg. 2014;23(2):273–8. https://doi.org/10.1016/j.jse.2013.09.026.
26. Ruch DS, Poehling GG. Anterior interosseus nerve injury following elbow arthroscopy. Arthroscopy. 1997;13(6):756–8.
27. Thomas MA, Fast A, Shapiro D. Radial nerve damage as a complication of elbow arthroscopy. Clin Orthop Relat Res. 1987;215:130–1.
28. Adams JE, Wolff LH 3rd, Merten SM, Steinmann SP. Osteoarthritis of the elbow: results of arthroscopic osteophyte resection and capsulectomy. J Shoulder Elb Surg. 2008;17(1):126–31. https://doi.org/10.1016/j.jse.2007.04.005.
29. Goyal D, Keyhani S, Lee EH, Hui JH. Evidence-based status of microfracture technique: a systematic review of level I and II studies. Arthroscopy. 2013;29(9):1579–88. https://doi.org/10.1016/j.arthro.2013.05.027.
30. Lubowitz JH. Arthroscopic microfracture may not be superior to arthroscopic debridement, but abrasion arthroplasty results are good, although not great. Arthroscopy. 2015;31(3):506. https://doi.org/10.1016/j.arthro.2015.01.004.
31. Menth-Chiari WA, Ruch DS, Poehling GG. Arthroscopic excision of the radial head: Clinical outcome in 12 patients with post-traumatic arthritis after fracture of the radial head or rheumatoid arthritis. Arthroscopy. 2001;17(9):918–23. https://doi.org/10.1053/jars.2001.28929.

Arthrofibrosis

9

Stefan Greiner

Contents

9.1 Pathology

Posttraumatic restricted mobility is one of the most common complications after elbow injuries or surgeries. The loss of full range of movement in the elbow leads to restrictions on activities of daily living such as body hygiene, eating, or using the phone. Restriction of the extension can lead to problems in reaching or positioning objects [1].

A study on 25 patients showed that there is an improvement in the range of motion 1 year after posttraumatic mobility restrictions in the elbow joint. In this study, only 12% of the patients had to undergo surgery for residual stiffness. However, the authors were able to show that a stagnation in the improvement in the range of motion 3 months after the trauma is an indication of an impending, treatment-resistant arthrofibrosis [2].

Kay classified posttraumatic elbow stiffness into five different entities based on the affected components [3]:

- Soft tissue contracture.
- Soft tissue contracture with ossifications.
- Nondisplaced articular fracture with soft tissue contractures.
- Dislocated intraarticular fracture with soft tissue contractures.
- Posttraumatic bony blockages.

The Morrey classification, on the other hand, is based more on the anatomical region that leads to the contracture; a distinction is made between intrinsic and extrinsic elbow stiffness [4]:

S. Greiner (✉)
Sporthopaedicum Regensburg-Straubing, Regensburg, Germany
e-mail: greiner@sporthopaedicum.de

A. B. Imhoff, A. Lenich (eds.), *Elbow Arthroscopy and Minimal Invasive Surgery*,
https://doi.org/10.1007/978-3-031-75611-5_9

Intrinsic factors (intraarticular changes):

- Free joint loose bodies.
- Synovitis.
- Intraarticular blockages.
- Osteoarthritis.

Extrinsic factors (extraarticular changes):

- Skin/soft tissue contractures.
- Capsular contractures.
- Ligament contractures.
- Heterotopic ossifications.
- Combination of intrinsic and extrinsic factors.

Primary arthrofibrosis involves massive connective tissue formation and generalized scarring of the capsular tissue of the elbow joint, the origin of which has not yet been clearly clarified. Both the cellular (increased number of myofibroblasts) and the extracellular matrix (increased collagen, disorganized fibers, collagen crosslinking, decreased proteoglycans, increased matrix metalloproteinases (MMP), and decreased tissue inhibitors of the MMP-related components) are possible causes that lead to capsular contracture [5, 6].

The remodeling is most likely impaired in the context of physiological wound healing. There is a dysregulation among mast cells, myofibroblasts, and neuropeptides (ketotifen, substance P) that leads to fibrosis [7]. This means that the balance between pro- and anti-inflammatory cytokines is mixed up in favor of the anti-inflammatory cytokine reactions, and the result is impaired wound healing with excessive scarring and irreversible tissue fibrosis.

9.2 Indication

In principle, the treatment of elbow joint arthrofibrosis should start with conservative therapy. The focus here is on a corresponding analgesic therapy in combination with the pain-adapted physiotherapeutic mobilization of the joint. Forced and repetitive mobilization are contraindicated, as this could intensify the existing clinical picture and favor on the contrary, as in animal experiments, the formation of heterotopic ossification [8].

A failed conservative therapy is therefore the main cause of the indication of an operative intervention. The period in which this conservative therapy is carried out, a period of 3 months, is an indicator of a therapy-resistant course [2].

According to Morrey, a range of motion of 100° (0–30–130° according to the neutral-zero method) in terms of extension and flexion, along with 50° pronation and supination each, is sufficient to cover 90% of the activities of daily life [4]. However, it must be taken into account that for many special activities, both at work and in leisure, a restricted range of motion of 100° is a clear obstacle and is associated with a significant loss of performance.

Basically, the treatment strategy is based on the symptoms and requirements of the patient, their level of activity, and the underlying cause of the contracture. The therapeutic options range from conservative therapy to open and arthroscopic arthrolysis techniques, interposition arthroplasty, partial or complete endoprosthetic joint replacement, and distraction arthroplasty [5, 9].

A prerequisite for performing arthroscopic arthrolysis is primarily intraarticular pathology. The simple, primarily intraarticular stiffness is the main indication for arthroscopic elbow joint arthrolysis.

9.3 Operating Principle/Instruments

The principle of operation initially involves the resection of bony blockages (osteophytes, free joint loose bodies) in the dorsal and ventral compartments. Furthermore, depending on the extent of the capsular contracture, a capsulectomy of the ventral and/or dorsal joint capsule must be performed to generate a satisfying surgical result. Microfracturing of areas with damaged articular cartilage is also recommended. Frayed and broken cartilage should be smoothed to form stable walls.

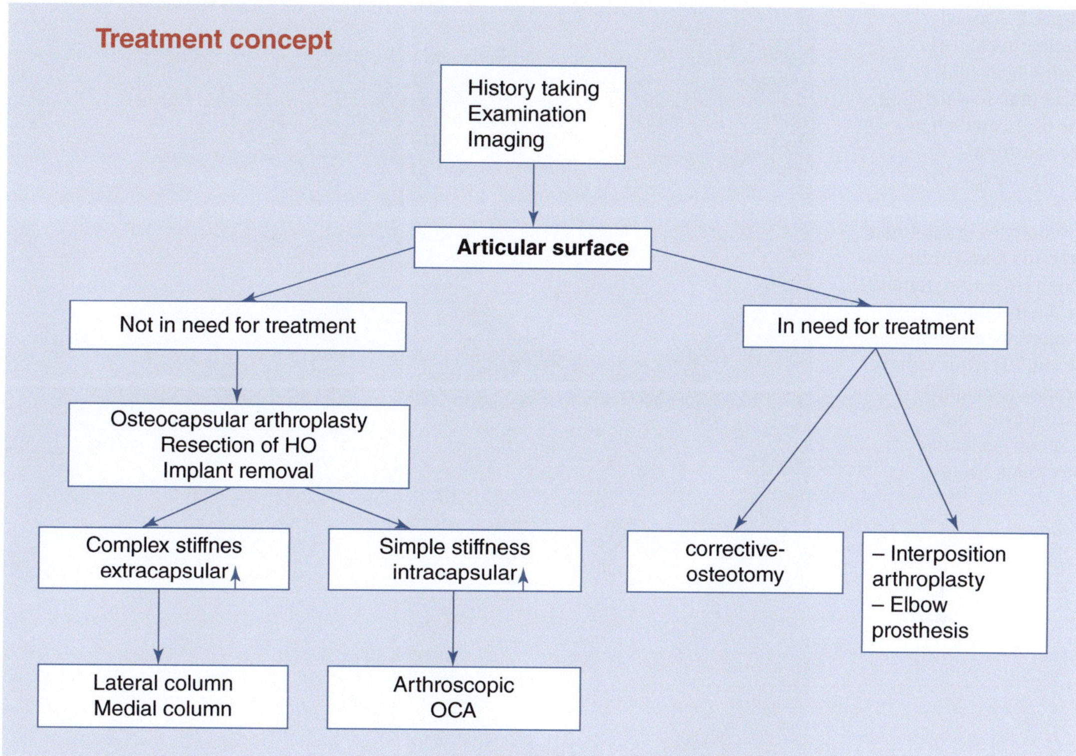

Fig. 9.1 Treatment concept. *HO* heterotopic ossifications, *OCA* osteocapsular arthroplasty

In addition to standard arthroscopic instruments, small chisels, retractors, awls with different curvatures for possible microfracturing, curettes, and small dissecting scissors are required to perform elbow joint arthrolysis (Fig. 9.1).

9.4 Surgical Technique

A dorsoventral approach is generally recommended, as different entities in both compartments will require treatment.

Dorsal Access

- Posterolateral.
- Posterior central.
- Soft spot, here possibly a high and a lower one.
- Soft-spot portal, especially in the case of osteochondrosis dissecans of the capitulum.
- Open neurolysis of the ulnar nerve. If necessary, release of the posterior bundle of the medial collateral ligament (pMCL).

Anterior Access

Anteroradial, anteroulnar, and additional portals may be needed for retractors to improve vision and protect soft tissue structures.

The following interventions should be performed dorsally (Fig. 9.2):

- Synovitis: Synovectomy with the shaver or the electrocautery.
- Osteophytes/free loose bodies: Removal of osteophytes with a chisel and removal of free loose bodies.
- Capsule (Fig. 9.3): Dorsal capsule release, paying attention to the ulnar nerve in the ulnar recess.

Range of motion test (ROM; no manipulation): After the end of the dorsal intervention, the range of motion that has been achieved is tested. Forced manipulation should be avoided. This can also be done under arthroscopic view via the posterolateral portal to avoid any remaining osseous impingement due to osteophytic attachments.

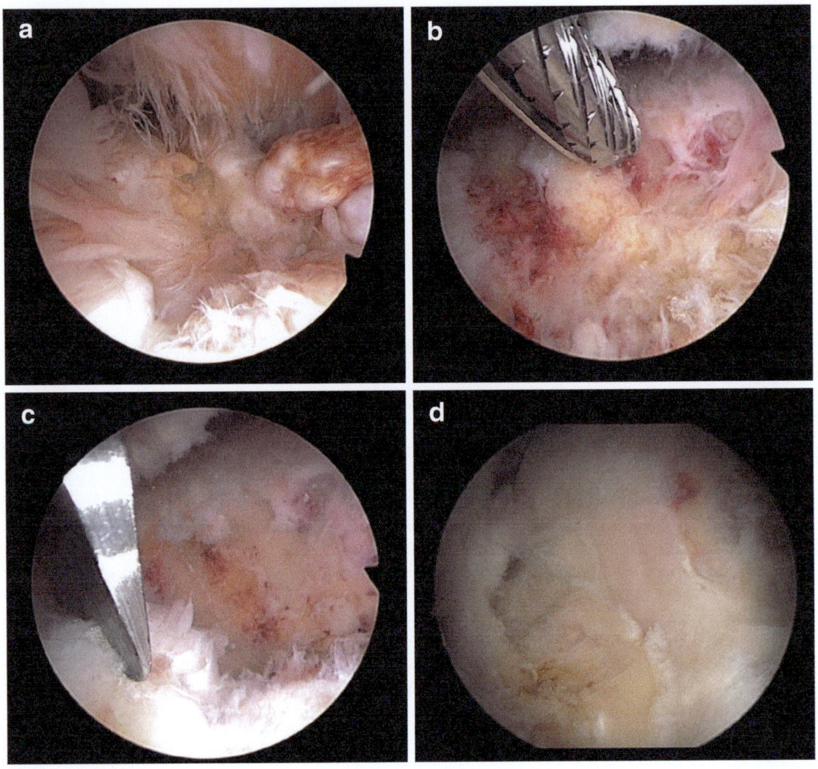

Fig. 9.2 Dorsal compartment. (**a**) Osteophytes in the olecranon fossa and on the olecranon when viewed from posterolateral. (**b**) Removal of the osteophytes in the fossa with the burr. (**c**) In slight extension, removal of the olecranon osteophytes with the chisel. (**d**) After removal of the olecranon osteophytes and osteophytes in the olecranon fossa

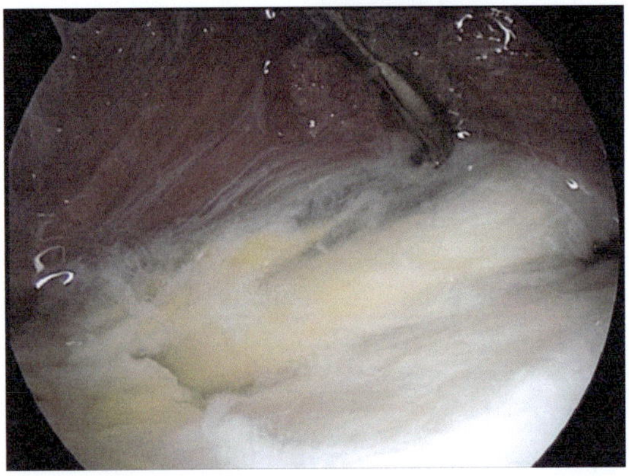

Fig. 9.3 After removal of the dorsal capsule, the ulnar nerve lies directly on the medial edge of the triceps

After that change to the ventral compartment takes place. The surgeon first goes into the joint with the camera via the anteroradial portal.

Ventral

Synovitis: Synovectomy with the shaver and the electrocautery.

Osteophytes/free loose bodies on the ulnar side: Viewed from the radial side and removal of osteophytes and free loose bodies.

Capsule (Fig. 9.4): The ulnar capsule is then freed. This can be done by first incising the capsule with small dissecting scissors. Then, the capsule edges are removed with the shaver.

Osteophytes/free loose bodies on the radial side: Now, the optic is changed to an anteroulnar portal. The remaining osteophytes and any free loose bodies are removed via the anteroradial portal.

Capsule (Fig. 9.5): Corresponding to the ulnar procedure, the final removal of the radial capsule takes place. The deep branch of the radial nerve, which is anterior to the head of the radius under the radial edge of the brachialis, should be spared here.

Finally, the mobility is tested again. Forced manipulation should not follow!

- Remaining flexion deficit: Possibly open release of the pMCL.

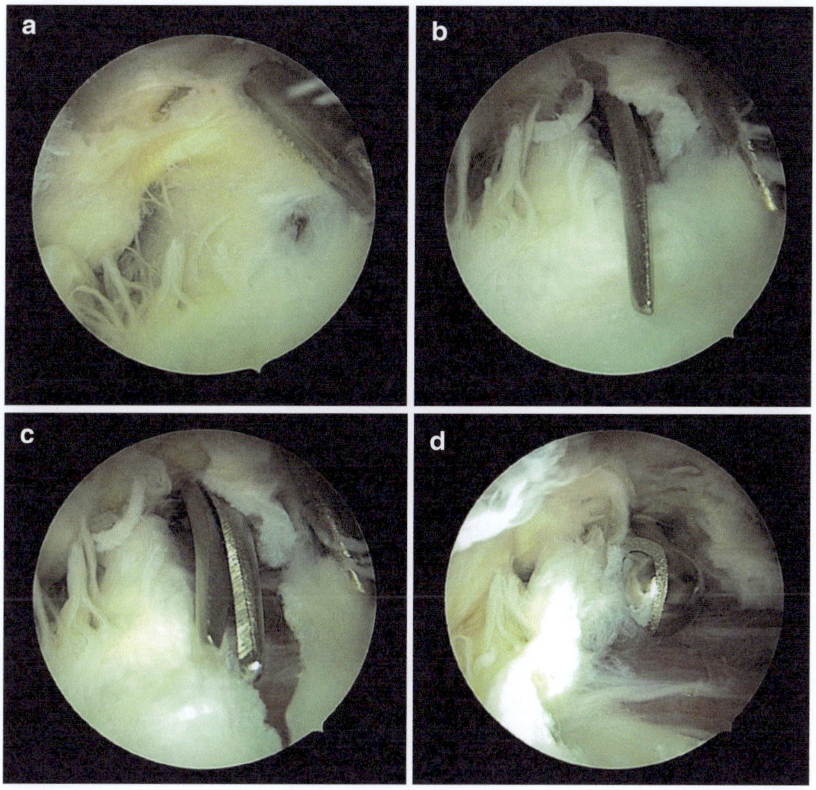

Fig. 9.4 (**a**) Viewing from the anteroradial portal showing the clearly thickened capsule. This is held with a switching stick or retractor to create space for the release of the ventral capsule. (**b**) The capsule is incised through the anteroulnar portal with dissecting scissors. (**c**) The brachialis muscle can be seen under the capsule. (**d**) The capsule edges can now be removed with the shaver

- Remaining extension deficit: Do complete ventral release.
- Dorsal osseous impingement.

Tips

- General: Large incisions: Better fluid extravasation.
- Always follow these rules:

1. Visibility: Only operate when visibility is assured.
2. Workplace: It is important to work in a sufficient space to be able to perform the surgical steps. The introduction of retractors is very helpful here!
3. Pay attention to neurovascular structures.

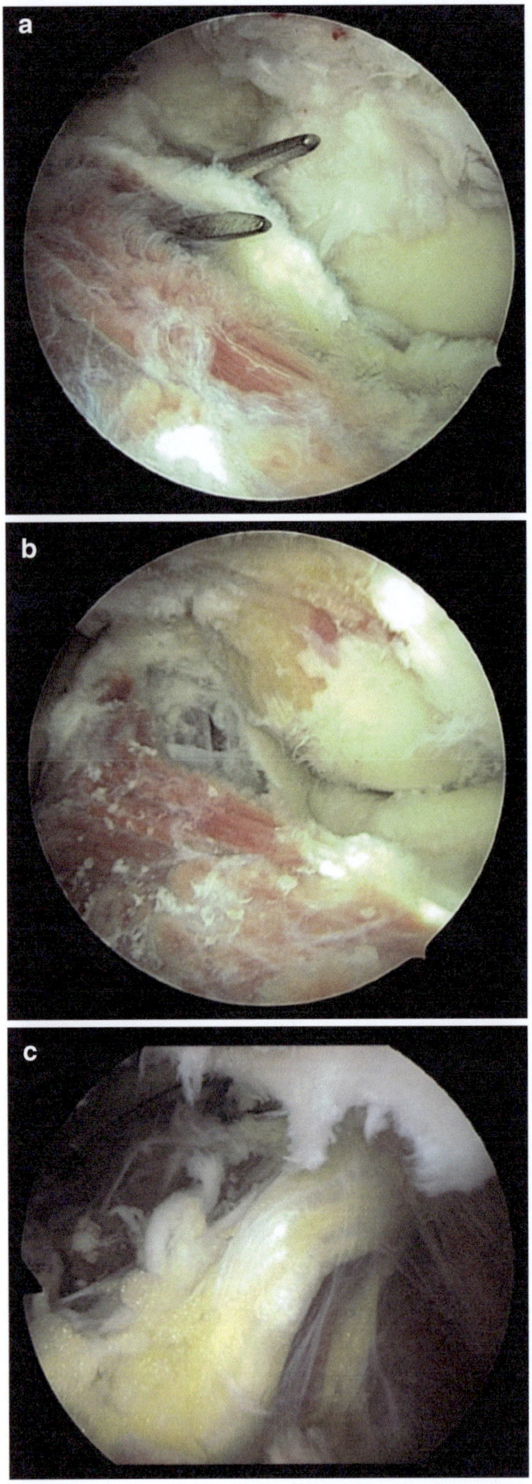

Fig. 9.5 (**a**) Change of optic to the anteroulnar portal and completion of the capsule release from the radial side. (**b**) Status after complete ventral release with exposed brachialis muscle. (**c**) If the brachialis muscle is pulled towards the ulnar side, the deep branch of the radial nerve becomes visible under its radial edge

9.5 Postoperative Measures

- Regardless of the preoperative range of motion, the author recommends the application of a ventral splint in full extension. This results in a compression of the ventral compartment and thus a reduction in bleeding. The splint is taken off during the day to practice the elbow exercises and applied again for the first ten nights postoperatively.
- Continuous passive motion (CPM).
- Physiotherapy.
- If necessary, bracing with splints to keep the joint in maximum flexion or extension for some time.
- Early control/intervention.
- If necessary, heterotopic ossification (HO) prophylaxis.

References

1. Murray MR, Saltzman MD, Gryzlo SM, Terry MA, Woodward CC, Nuber GW. Efficacy of preoperative home use of 2% chlorhexidine gluconate cloth before shoulder surgery. J Shoulder Elb Surg. 2011;20(6):928–33. https://doi.org/10.1016/j.jse.2011.02.018.
2. Myden C, Hildebrand K. Elbow joint contracture after traumatic injury. J Shoulder Elb Surg. 2011;20(1):39–44.
3. Kay NR. Surgery of the elbow. London: Arnold; 1998.
4. Morrey BF. Post-traumatic contracture of the elbow. Operative treatment, including distraction arthroplasty. J Bone Joint Surg Am. 1990;72(4):601–18.
5. Charalambous CP, Morrey BF. Posttraumatic elbow stiffness. J Bone Joint Surg. 2012;94(15):1428–37. https://doi.org/10.2106/JBJS.K.00711.
6. Monument MJ, Hart DA, Salo PT, Befus AD, Hildebrand KA. Posttraumatic elbow contractures: targeting neuroinflammatory fibrogenic mechanisms. J Orthop Sci. 2013;18(6):869–77.
7. Hildebrand KA. Posttraumatic elbow joint contractures: defining pathologic capsular mechanisms and potential future treatment paradigms. J Hand Surg Am. 2013;38(11):2227–33.
8. Lindenhovius ALC, Jupiter JB. The posttraumatic stiff elbow: a review of the literature. J Hand Surg Am. 2007;32(10):1605–23.
9. Everding N, Maschke S, Hoyen H, Evans P. Prevention and treatment of elbow stiffness: a 5-year update. J Hand Surg Am. 2013;38(12):2496–507.

Endoscopic Neurolysis and Transposition of the Ulnar Nerve

10

Andreas Lenich

Contents

10.1 Introduction

Due to its exposed position, the ulnar nerve is predisposed to injuries. The secondary consequences, such as restricted mobility of the elbow joint or pain, can often only be recognized as ulnar nerve complaints due to the closer proximity of the ulnar nerve, and this can be diagnosed by clinical examination.

The ulnar nerve pathologies can be differentiated into intrinsic and extrinsic. With the exception of the swelling of the nerves as an intrinsic cause, only the extrinsic causes are accessible to endoscopic therapy and are described here [1].

A. Lenich (✉)
ZEST – Zentrum for Elbow and Shoulder Therapy, Munich, Germany

10.2 Pathology

When the elbow is flexed at 90°, the space around the nerve in the area of the ulnar groove is reduced with a reduction in diameter of about 50%. Extrinsic pathologies such as hematomas, scars, osteophytes, or intrinsic pathologies can lead to swelling of the nerve in the constriction areas and thus limit its mobility. This narrowness leads to a reflex tension in the antagonistic muscles, which leads to a reduction in the range of motion of the elbow joint [1]. The nerve conduction velocity is measured as standard with an extended arm and does not change noticeably in this pathological form of the ulnar nerve constriction. Reduced measurement results can only be documented in case of nerve damage or if the measurement is

A. B. Imhoff, A. Lenich (eds.), *Elbow Arthroscopy and Minimal Invasive Surgery*,
https://doi.org/10.1007/978-3-031-75611-5_10

done while the elbow is in flexion and the shoulder is in abduction.

10.3 Diagnosis

10.3.1 Medical History

A trauma history with specific inquiries to the elbow should be documented. Paresthesia of the little and ulnar side of the ring finger and/or loss of strength in the hypothenar area.

10.3.2 Clinical Evaluation

Due to its superficial course, the ulnar nerve in the area of the elbow can be accessible to direct palpation. A jumping/snapping nerve may be noticed when moving the elbow. Sensation deficits in the little finger and the ring finger on the ulnar side are recorded using a 2-point discrimination test (sharp pointed and stump object). The Hoffmann–Tinel test can be checked in the area of the ulnar groove and Guyon canal.

10.3.3 Diagnostic Imaging

Sonography
The ultrasound examination of the ulnar nerve allows a static as well as a dynamic examination. Most of the constrictions can be shown very well. With the static examination technique, the nerve can be shown as hourglass-shaped constrictions. In the dynamic examination, the lack of gliding is noticeable in the case of a fixed nerve.

Conventional X-Ray Diagnostics
The X-rays of the elbow joint in anteroposterior (a.p.) and laterally are the standard images. Ulnar groove view can reveal osseous changes such as constrictions due to osteophytes.

Sectional Image Diagnostics
A CT examination of the elbow joint is indicated if there is any suspicion of osseous changes in the area of the ulnar groove to precisely localize them preoperatively.

The course of the nerve and its accompanying soft tissue structures can be shown using MRI. Constrictions due to swellings, tumors, scarring, and hematomas, as well as deviations from the normal course, can be also shown in MRI.

10.4 Indications for Surgery

Endoscopic decompression of the ulnar nerve is indicated for extrinsic constriction due to fibrous tissue, hematoma, or defects in the fascia [2, 3].

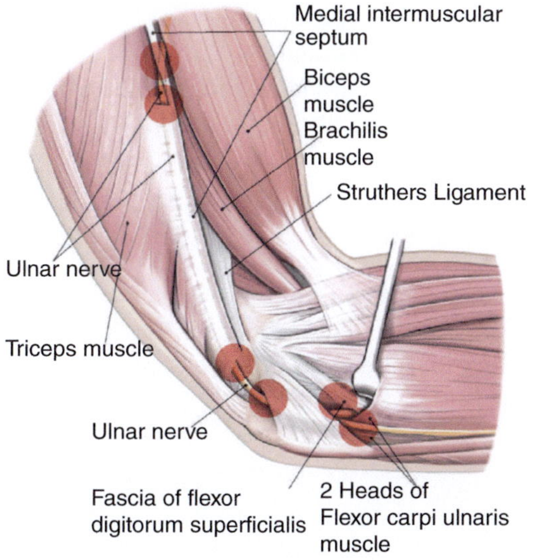

Fig. 10.1 Physiological constrictions in the course of the ulnar nerve near the elbow joint

10.5 Principle of Operation/ Instruments

A distinction must be made between open and endoscopic neurolysis. Standard surgical instruments can be used for open neurolysis. Endoscopic neurolysis has the advantage of the small skin incision length. For endoscopic neurolysis, special instruments are required to enable subcutaneous tunneling (forceps/speculum) and endoscopic decompression of the nerve (special nerve trocar for the optics/long fine dissecting scissors) (Figs. 10.1 and 10.2).

10.6 Preparation for the Surgery

Previous operations and injuries must be taken into account, especially previous decompression attempts. The patient must be informed about the extensive follow-up treatment. A plexus catheter is applied preoperatively but is only used postoperatively after the nerve functions have been checked and documented.

In case of isolated nerve decompression, the patient is placed on his back with his arm extended on the hand table. A tourniquet is applied, but it is not absolutely necessary.

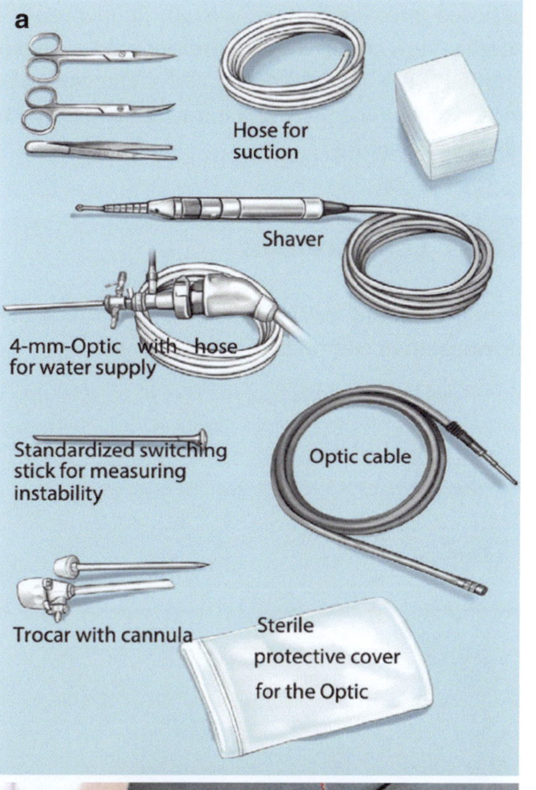

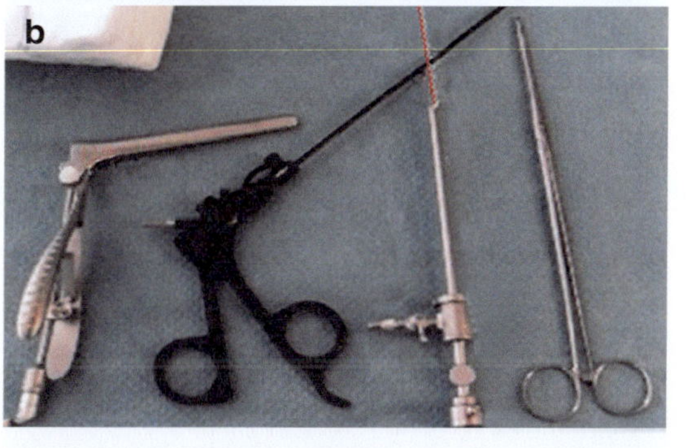

Fig. 10.2 (**a**) Instruments for endoscopic neurolysis. (**b**) Instruments from left to right: Speculum, trocar with soft tissue sleeve, forceps (Storz or Wolf)

10.7 Surgical Technique

Endoscopic neurolysis of the ulnar nerve begins with a medial skin incision in the area of the ulnar groove. After displaying the nerves in the groove, use the forceps to create a subcutaneous tunnel proximally and distally in the assumed nerve course. This tunnel is expanded with the speculum and serves as a working space for the endoscope. With dissecting scissors, the nerve is exposed proximally and distally under endoscopic view until all constrictions have been splitted (Figs. 10.3, 10.4, and 10.5). The wound is closed subcutaneously and intracutaneously with absorbable sutures.

10.7.1 Complications

Patients should be informed of the following postoperative complications [4–6]:

- Irreparable nerve lesion.
- Temporary paresthesia.
- Increasing restricted mobility of the elbow.
- General surgical complications.

10.7.2 Results

The study of endoscopic versus open neurolysis of the ulnar nerve by Fowler's group shows that the endoscopic technique is superior [3].

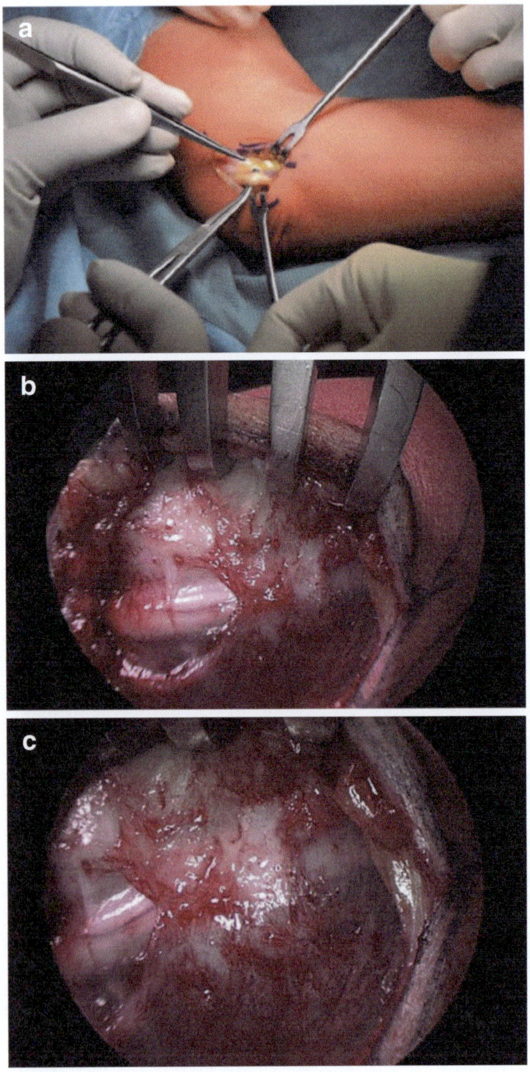

Fig. 10.3 (a–c) Approach

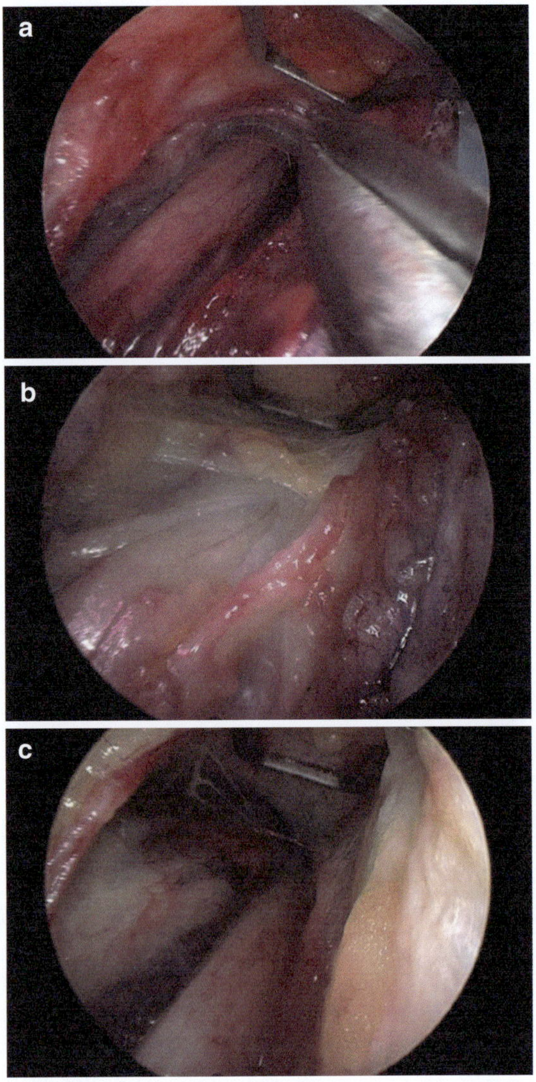

Fig. 10.4 (a–c) Endoscopic dissection in the distal direction

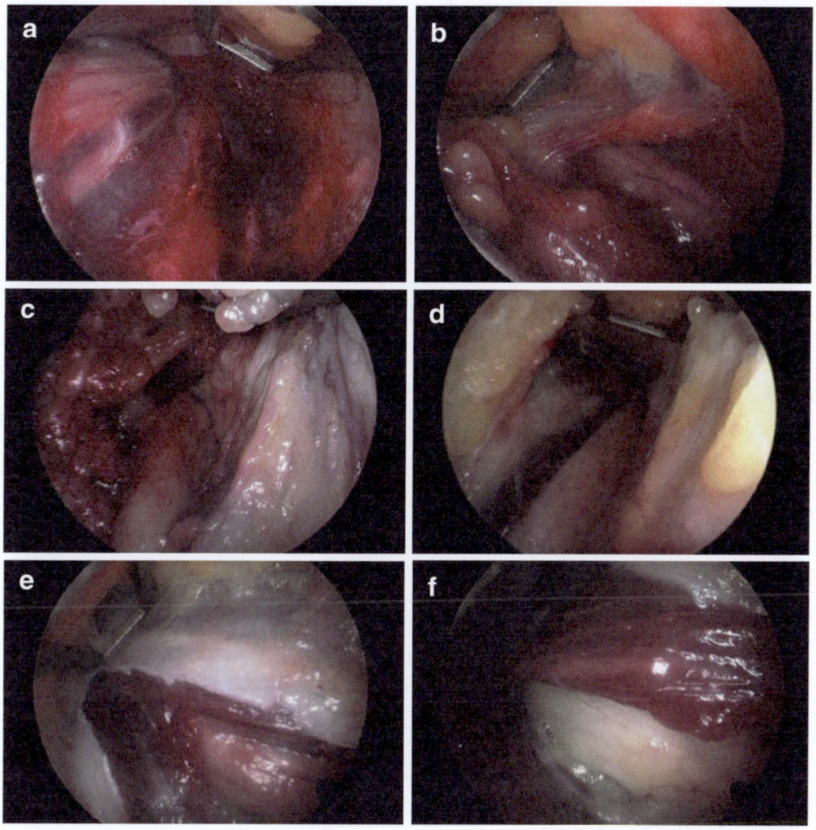

Fig. 10.5 (a–f) Endoscopic dissection in the proximal direction

10.8 Postoperative Measures

After the anesthesia has ended, the ulnar nerve supply area should be checked immediately. The pain catheter can only be used with local anesthetic after a reliable neurological evaluation. Mobilization after operative arthrolysis, intensive physiotherapy, and exercise with continuous passive motion (CPM) for 6 weeks adequate with analgesic therapy is recommended (Fig. 10.6) [7].

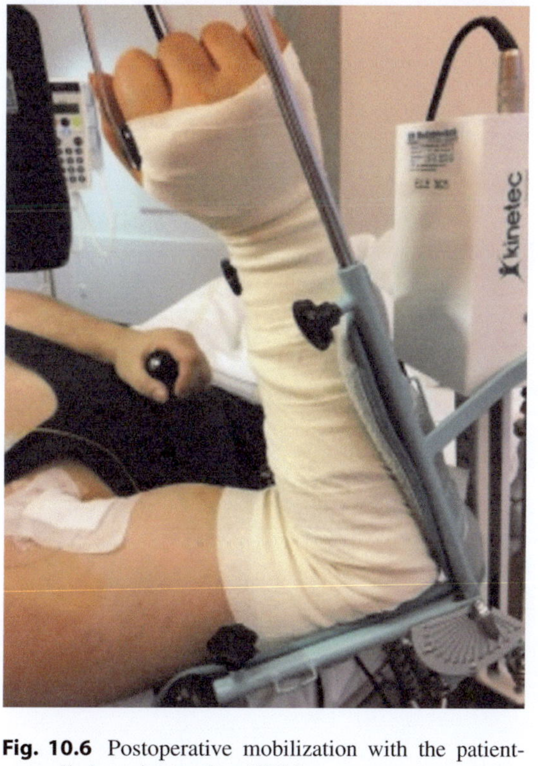

Fig. 10.6 Postoperative mobilization with the patient-controlled passive motion (CPM)

References

1. Eberlin KR, Marjoua Y, Jupiter JB. Compressive neuropathy of the ulnar nerve: a perspective on history and current controversies. J Hand Surg Am. 2017;42(6):464–9.
2. Morse LP, McGuire DT, Bain GI. Endoscopic ulnar nerve release and transposition. Tech Hand Up Extrem Surg. 2014;18(1):10–4.
3. Toirac A, Giugale JM, Fowler JR. Open versus endoscopic cubital tunnel in situ decompression: a systematic review of outcomes and complications. Hand (N Y). 2017;12(3):229–35.
4. Hamdi MF, Aloui I, Allagui M. Ulnar nerve compression at the elbow and heterotropic ossification: a report of five cases. Neurochirurgie. 2010;56:340–3.
5. Kelly EW, Morrey BF, O'Driscoll SW. Complications of elbow arthroscopy. J Bone Joint Surg Am. 2001;83A:25–34.
6. Prommersberger KJ, Mühldorfer M, van Schoonhoven J. Neurologische Komplikationen bei Ellenbogensteife. Orthopäde. 2011;40:323–7.
7. Lindenhovius AL, van de Luijtgaarden K, Ring D, et al. Open elbow contracture release: postoperative management with and without continuous passive motion. J Hand Surg Am. 2009;34A:858–65.

Endoscopically Assisted Refixation of the Distal Part of the Biceps Tendon

11

Andreas Lenich and Sven Reuter

Contents

11.1 Pathology/Indication

Most of the distal biceps tendon ruptures are directly related to an acute incident [1]. The combination of a sudden eccentric force acting on an actively flexed elbow is often the cause of a tendon rupture [2, 3]. The incidence of distal biceps tendon rupture is 1.2 ruptures per 100,000 inhabitants per year [4]. Men between the ages of 30 and 60 are particularly affected, with an increased incidence in the fourth and fifth decades of life [4].

A. Lenich (✉)
ZEST – Zentrum for Elbow and Shoulder Therapy, Munich, Germany

S. Reuter
University of Applied Health Sciences, Campus Stuttgart, Stuttgart, Germany
e-mail: info@prehabsportsmedicine.com

The indication for an operation in patients with an acute complete or partial rupture with significant loss of strength of supination and flexion of the elbow joint. Surgical reinsertion of the tendon in the radial tuberosity is currently considered as the standard procedure [2, 5]. There is a clear consensus that surgical therapy is superior to conservative therapy for regaining flexion and supination power in the elbow joint [2, 4, 6].

In recent years, various surgical techniques have been described to offer the optimal refixation method with good functional results. Nevertheless, both the operative approach (single-incision technique vs. double-incision technique) and the refixation method (suture anchor, endobutton, transosseous sutures, interference screw) are still controversial with regard to the optimal restoration of strength and the minimization of complications [7–9].

A. B. Imhoff, A. Lenich (eds.), *Elbow Arthroscopy and Minimal Invasive Surgery*,
https://doi.org/10.1007/978-3-031-75611-5_11

A frequently reported complication of the single-incision approach is the transient or persistent irritation of the lateral antebrachial cutaneous nerve due to the pulling effect of the hook or direct compression during the operation [10, 11]. To minimize this complication, endoscopically assisted techniques for refixing the distal biceps tendon have already been discussed [12, 13]. Biomechanical studies have shown that the exact anatomical reinsertion of the distal biceps tendon is crucial, and deviations of a few millimeters can result in a considerable reduction in the supination force [14, 15]. A precise intraoperative view of the radial tuberosity is, therefore, essential for implant placement, which can be facilitated by the endoscopic view.

11.2 Principle of Operation/ Instruments

In the technique presented here, the distal biceps tendon is reinserted at the radial tuberosity using intramedullary fixation plates through a minimally invasive, endoscopically assisted procedure. Searching for the tendon stump and preparing the radial tuberosity with the positioning of the drill holes under endoscopic control are essential for the success of the operation. The tendon stump is then anatomically intramedullary refixed in the radial tuberosity using two fixation plates.

Instruments

- 2 biceps buttons for intramedullary fixation (from Arthrex, Naples, FL, USA).
- 2× FiberWire 2.0 (from Arthrex, Naples, FL, USA).
- 2× 2.4-mm drill guide wires.
- Drill bit 3.2 mm (Acumed Ltd., Hempshire, UK).
- Protective sleeve 3.5 mm.
- Nerve preparation attachment for the endoscopic camera.

11.3 Preparations for Surgery

First, the medical history is taken with documentation of the course of symptoms after the injury, previous complaints and previous operations at the elbow, the preoperative neurovascular status must be documented. As part of the symptom-specific examination, attention must be paid to the proximalization of the muscle belly of the biceps brachii and the presence of hematoma around the elbow. A comparison of the muscle function test with the noninjured side often reveals a reduced force in supination and a positive hook test. An X-ray of the elbow in two planes (anteroposterior and lateral) and an MRI scan to assess the extent of the tendon damage (partial vs. complete), the level of the lesion, the tendon quality, and the assessment of the retraction of the tendon stump are done to complete the preoperative diagnosis.

In the patient's clarification, attention must be drawn to the risk of intraoperative nerve injuries (radial nerve, median nerve, musculocutaneous nerve), vascular injuries, and residual functional disorders. The formation of heterotopic ossifications and rerupture of the tendon are also possible complications that must be mentioned. In addition to the incorrect placement of the fixation systems, these systems can break out, loosen, or dislocate. The procedure is performed in a supine position under general anesthesia. The extremity to be operated on is positioned on a radiolucent arm table with the elbow extended and the forearm in a supination position. A tourniquet (280 mmHg) is applied.

11.4 Surgical Technique

The incision is made just distal to the elbow on the ulnar side (Fig. 11.1). The medial edge of the brachioradialis muscle serves as the guiding structure. The lateral cutaneous antebrachial nerve (the musculocutaneous nerve) must be spared in its course on the fascia of the brachioradialis. The fascia is incised just medial to the brachioradialis muscle.

The tendon stump, which is usually retracted proximally, is found with the endoscope (Fig. 11.2). Removal of the adhesions is carried out under vision. The radial tuberosity is palpated while the elbow is in flexion and supination position. The radial tuberosity is exposed and prepared under endoscopic visualization (Fig. 11.3).

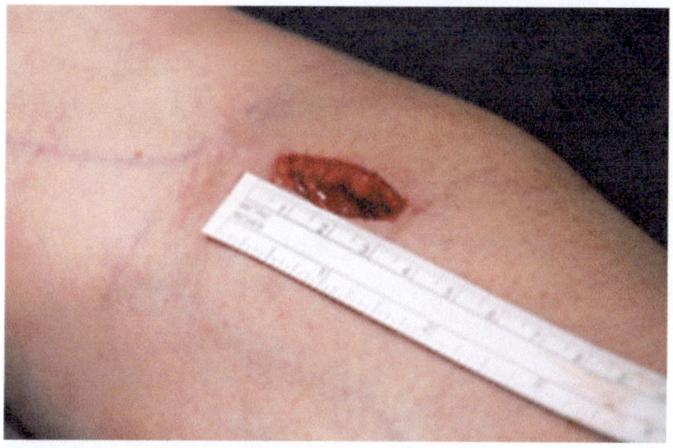

Fig. 11.1 Approach on the ulnar side of the elbow

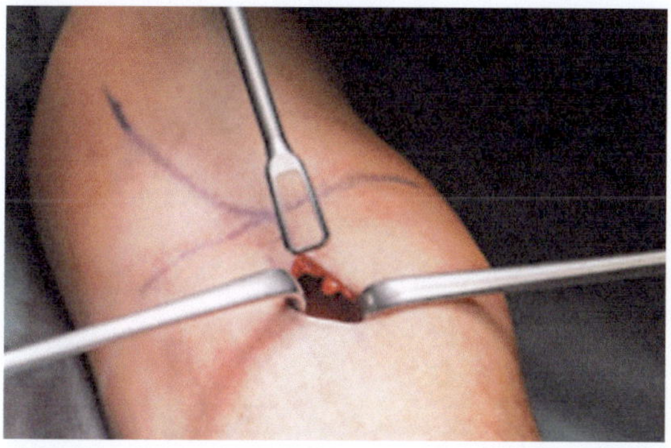

Fig. 11.2 Entrance with the endoscope (with nerve preparation attachment)

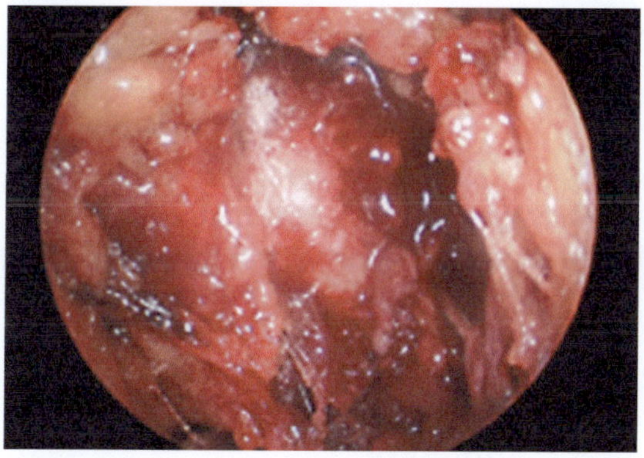

Fig. 11.3 Preparation of the radial tuberosity

The tendon stump is looped with non-resorbable suture material (e.g., FiberWire, Arthrex) with an ascending Krakow suture beginning at the distal end and then descending toward the opposite tendon edge. Two pairs of threads are placed on the tendon stump (Fig. 11.4). Each pair of threads is then loaded with a biceps button (Fig. 11.5).

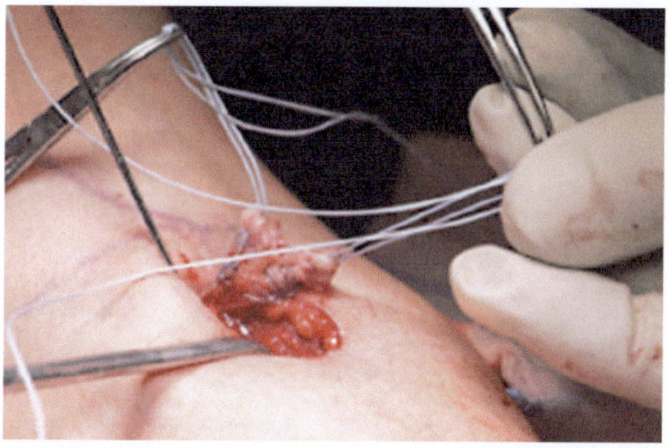

Fig. 11.4 Tying the tendon stump with two pairs of sutures

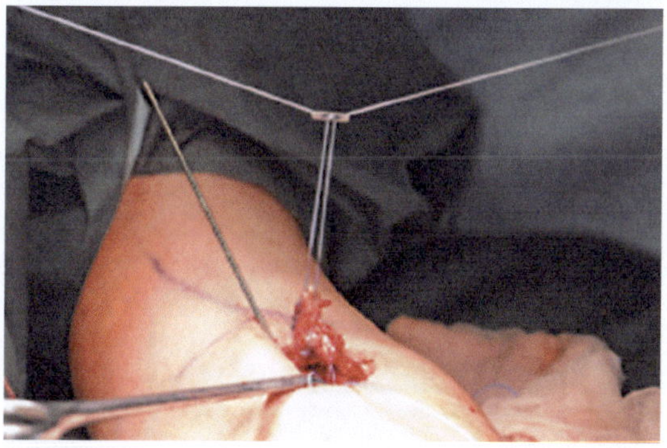

Fig. 11.5 Attaching the sutures pairs with two biceps buttons

With the forearm in the maximum supination position, two guide wires are placed in the radial tuberosity, and the correct placement of the drill wires is then checked radiologically by the C-Arm (Fig. 11.6). A drill sleeve is now placed over the wires, and the guide wire is removed. The 3.2-mm drill is then used to drill only the near cortex to the opposite cortex without penetrating it. The biceps buttons are inserted into the respective drill hole one after the other and pushed forward subcortically until they tilt (Fig. 11.7). Pulling on the free threads ensures that both buttons are "flipped" into the intramedullary subcortex of the near cortex. Then, the thread ends are knotted.

Finally, the buttons' positions are checked radiologically in two planes, and the free passive mobility of the joint is also checked (Fig. 11.8).

Tips and Tricks

During the deep preparation and placement of the drill holes, the forearm should be placed in maxi-

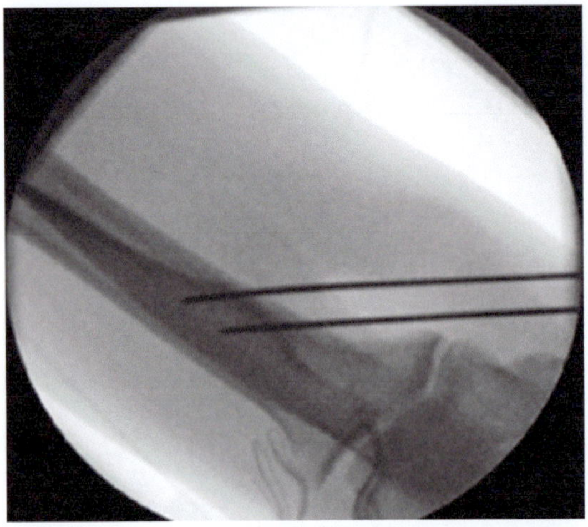

Fig. 11.6 Radiological control of the guide wire position in the radial tuberosity

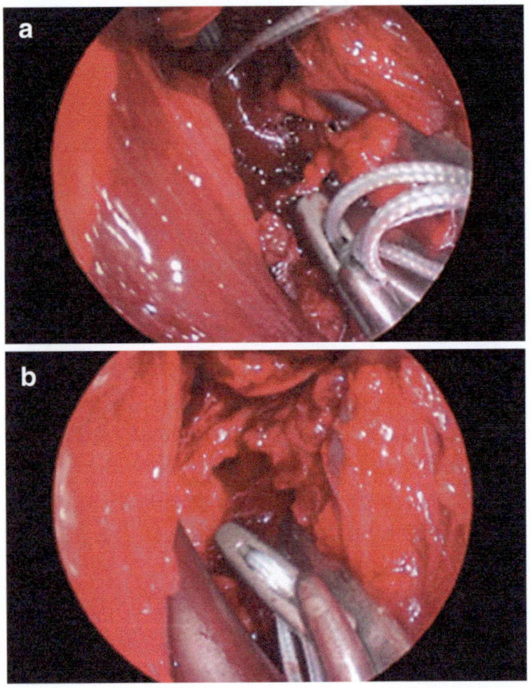

Fig. 11.7 (**a**, **b**) Insertion of the two biceps buttons in the drill holes and subcortical flipping

mum supination to achieve the anatomical reinsertion of the tendon. In addition, after the drilling of the tunnels, extensive irrigation should be carried out to prevent the development of heterotopic ossifications postoperatively. The recurrent rami of the perforating veins must be ligated carefully to prevent bleeding. In order not to endanger the pull-out stability of the buttons, no extensive debridement should be performed in the cortical region.

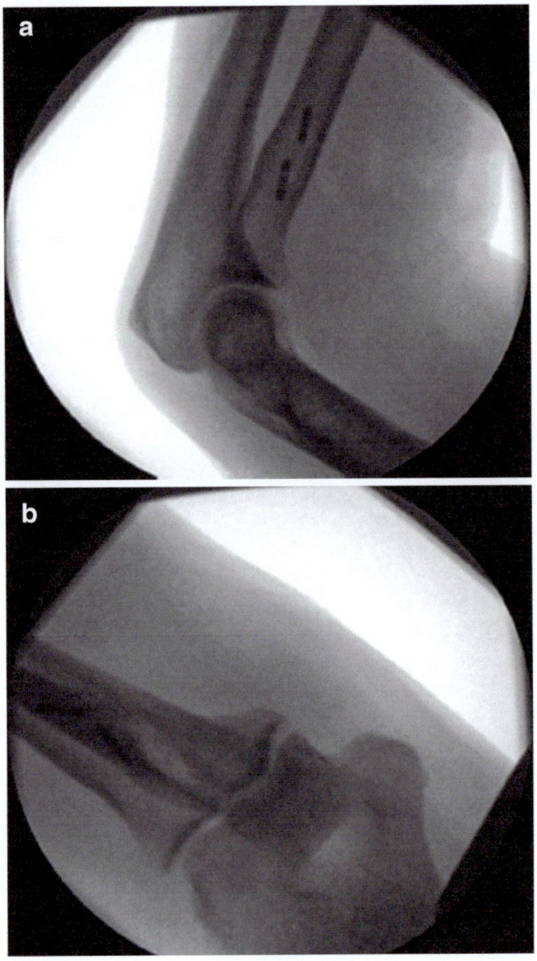

Fig. 11.8 (**a**, **b**) Final radiological checkup

11.5 Summary

Objective of the operation: Endoscopically assisted refixation of the distal biceps tendon at the radial tuberosity with two buttons placed intramedullary subcortically.

Indications: Acute complete or partial ruptures of the distal biceps tendon with significant loss of strength for supination and flexion in the elbow joint.

Surgical technique: Skin incision is done just distal to the elbow on the ulnar side. Examination with the endoscope is carried out. Search for the tendon stump and endoscopic exposure of the radial tuberosity. Sling the tendon stump with two pairs of threads, which are then loaded with two biceps buttons. After placing two guide wires in the radial tuberosity and over-drilling is carried out, the buttons are placed subcortically and flipped intramedullary.

11.6 Postoperative Measures

There is an early functional follow-up treatment with free passive mobilization.

An EpicoROM® orthosis (from Medi, Bayreuth, Germany) is worn for a total period of 6 weeks.

In the orthosis, the extension is limited to 20° for 4 weeks. In addition, no active pronation/supination is allowed in the first 2 weeks postoperatively.

Maximum sports activity and hard physical work are possible again after 12 weeks. Active biceps activities with weights >5 kg should be avoided for 6 weeks.

References

1. Klonz A, Loitz D, Reilmann H. Proximal and distal ruptures of the biceps brachii tendon. Unfallchirurg. 2003;106(9):755–63.
2. Chillemi C, Marinelli M, De Cupis V. Rupture of the distal biceps brachii tendon: conservative treatment versus anatomic reinsertion – clinical and radiological evaluation after 2 years. Arch Orthop Trauma Surg. 2007;127(8):705–8. https://doi.org/10.1007/s00402-007-0326-7.
3. Hegelmaier C, Schramm W, Lange P. Distal biceps tendon rupture. Therapy and forensic insurance evaluation. Unfallchirurg. 1992;95(1):9–16.
4. Morrey ME, Abdel MP, Sanchez-Sotelo J, Morrey BF. Primary repair of retracted distal biceps tendon ruptures in extreme flexion. J Shoulder Elbow Surg/Am Shoulder Elbow Surg. 2014;23(5):679–85. https://doi.org/10.1016/j.jse.2013.12.030.
5. Bak K, Haugegaard LM, Petersen OC. Complete restoration of supination and flexion strength after surgical treatment of distal biceps tendon rupture by the Boyd-Andersson method. Ugesk Laeger. 1992;154(10):629–31.
6. Nesterenko S, Domire ZJ, Morrey BF, Sanchez-Sotelo J. Elbow strength and endurance in patients with a ruptured distal biceps tendon. J Shoulder Elbow Surg/Am Shoulder Elbow Surg. 2010;19(2):184–9. https://doi.org/10.1016/j.jse.2009.06.001.
7. Hartman MW, Merten SM, Steinmann SP. Mini-open 2-incision technique for repair of distal biceps tendon ruptures. J Shoulder Elbow Surg/Am Shoulder Elbow Surg. 2007;16(5):616–20. https://doi.org/10.1016/j.jse.2006.10.021.
8. Hasan SA, Cordell CL, Rauls RB, Bailey MS, Sahu D, Suva LJ. Two-incision versus one-incision repair for distal biceps tendon rupture: a cadaveric study. J Shoulder Elbow Surg/Am Shoulder Elbow Surg. 2012;21(7):935–41. https://doi.org/10.1016/j.jse.2011.04.027.
9. Watson JN, Moretti VM, Schwindel L, Hutchinson MR. Repair techniques for acute distal biceps tendon ruptures: a systematic review. J Bone Joint Surg Am. 2014;96(24):2086–90. https://doi.org/10.2106/JBJS.M.00481.
10. Grewal R, Athwal GS, MacDermid JC, et al. Single versus double-incision technique for the repair of acute distal biceps tendon ruptures: a randomized clinical trial. J Bone Joint Surg Am. 2012;94(13):1166–74. https://doi.org/10.2106/JBJS.K.00436.
11. Shields E, Olsen JR, Williams RB, Rouse L, Maloney M, Voloshin I. Distal biceps brachii tendon repairs: a single-incision technique using a cortical button with interference screw versus a double-incision technique using suture fixation through bone tunnels. Am J Sports Med. 2015;43(5):1072–6. https://doi.org/10.1177/0363546515570465.
12. Gregory T, Roure P, Fontes D. Repair of distal biceps tendon rupture using a suture anchor: description of a new endoscopic procedure. Am J Sports Med. 2009;37(3):506–11. https://doi.org/10.1177/0363546508326985.
13. Sharma S, MacKay G. Endoscopic repair of distal biceps tendon using an EndoButton. Arthroscopy. 2005;21(7):897. https://doi.org/10.1016/j.arthro.2005.04.001.
14. Bain GI, Prem H, Heptinstall RJ, Verhellen R, Paix D. Repair of distal biceps tendon rupture: a new technique using the Endobutton. J Shoulder Elbow Surg/Am Shoulder Elbow Surg. 2000;9(2):120–6.
15. Hutchinson HL, Gloystein D, Gillespie M. Distal biceps tendon insertion: an anatomic study. J Shoulder Elbow Surg/Am Shoulder Elbow Surg. 2008;17(2):342–6. https://doi.org/10.1016/j.jse.2007.05.005.

Arthroscopically Assisted Fracture Treatment

12

Lars P. Müller, Michael Hackl, Kilian Wegmann, and George S. Athwal

Contents

L. P. Müller (✉) · M. Hackl
Department of Orthopedic and Trauma Surgery, University Hospital of Cologne, Cologne, Germany
e-mail: lars.mueller@uk-koeln.de; michael.hackl@uk-koeln.de

K. Wegmann
OCM (Orthopädische Chirurgie München) Clinic, München, Germany
e-mail: kilian.wegmann@ocm-muenchen.de

G. S. Athwal
HULC, St. Joseph's Health Care, University of Western Ontario, London, ON, Canada
e-mail: gathwal@uwo.ca

12.1 Pathology

About 5–8% of all fractures in adults involve the elbow joint [1]. Persistent complaints are not uncommon. Particularly, after elbow dislocation and distal humerus fractures, they are often complicated with secondary osteoarthritis [2–4].

12.1.1 Frontal Shear Fractures of the Distal Humerus

Frontal shear fractures of the capitulum or trochlea (AO type 13 B3) are in some cases amenable to

A. B. Imhoff, A. Lenich (eds.), *Elbow Arthroscopy and Minimal Invasive Surgery*,
https://doi.org/10.1007/978-3-031-75611-5_12

arthroscopically assisted osteosynthesis and were classified by Dubberley et al. [5] as follows:

- **Dubberley Type I**: Simple shear fracture of the capitulum with or without involvement of the lateral edge of the trochlea.
- **Dubberley Type II**: Simple shear fracture of the capitulum and trochlea.
- **Dubberley Type III**: Multifragment shear fracture of the capitulum and trochlea.

Depending on the presence of a dorsal comminution zone, it is an A fracture (no dorsal comminution zone) or B fracture (dorsal comminution zone).

Displaced fractures of the distal humerus are usually treated surgically. The results after conservative therapy are mostly unsatisfactory, which is why conservative treatment is reserved for multimorbid, geriatric patients with low functional demands [6–8].

12.1.2 Coronoid Fractures

The coronoid process makes a significant contribution to the stability of the elbow joint. The sublime tubercle serves as an attachment for the anterior bundle of the medial collateral ligament and thus plays an important role in valgus stability [9]. In addition, it stabilizes the elbow joint against varus loads and limits the posterolateral rotation [10, 11]. Isolated coronoid fractures are rare; they often occur as accompanying pathologies. Regan and Morrey classified the coronoid fractures into three types [12]:

- Regan/Morrey Type I: Coronoid tip fracture.
- Regan/Morrey Type II: Fracture of <50% of the coronoid.
- Regan/Morrey Type III: Fracture of >50% of the coronoid.

The anteromedial facet fractures in particular were subclassified by O'Driscoll [9]:

- Type 1: Isolated transverse fracture.
- Type 2: Fracture with involvement of the anteromedial facet.
- Type 3: Fracture with involvement of the sublime tubercle.

Type I fractures according to Regan and Morrey can be treated conservatively. If a surgical decision is made to address the coronoid fragment during the surgical treatment of accompanying pathologies, this can be indirectly fixed by tying the ventral capsule. For type II fractures and type III fractures, surgical intervention with screw or plate osteosynthesis is usually indicated.

12.1.3 Radial Head Fractures

Fractures of the radial head are the most common bony elbow injury in adults [13, 14]. They usually result from a fall on the pronated arm and are frequently associated with relevant accompanying injuries in the collateral ligaments, the interosseous membrane, and/or the coronoid process [15–18].

The fracture classification is based on the Mason classification modified by Johnston [13]:

- Mason I: Simple, non-dislocated fracture (<2 mm dislocation).
- Mason II: Simple, dislocated fracture (>2 mm dislocation).
- Mason III: Multifragment fracture.
- Mason IV: Fracture dislocation.

While non-displaced fractures are treated conservatively, close monitoring is necessary to discover the complications at an early stage [19]. In case of displaced fractures, osteosynthesis is usually indicated, which is carried out with cannulated headless compression screws or, if the neck of the radius is involved, with the anatomically preformed locked plate. The resection of the radius head in the acute situation should not be carried out because of the multiple accompanying pathologies that should be addressed too. From our point of view, a prosthetic replacement is therefore preferable only in non-reconstructible fractures [20].

12.2 Indication

The arthroscopically assisted osteosynthesis allows a dedicated assessment of the associated pathologies, in particular of the articular cartilage and the collateral ligaments, contrary to the open procedure, in which only some parts of the joint can be seen and thus the accompanying injuries may remain undetected. In addition, the anatomical fracture reduction and the positioning of the osteosynthesis material can be verified arthroscopically, which reduces the need for intraoperative fluoroscopy.

The minimally invasive procedure also offers the advantage of lower morbidity and can thus potentially reduce the risk of pseudarthrosis, postoperative arthrofibrosis, or heterotopic ossification [21, 22].

The following types of fractures are suitable for arthroscopically assisted osteosynthesis:

- B3 fractures of the distal humerus without relevant comminution (Dubberley IA, IIA).
- Coronoid fractures without relevant comminution (Regan/Morrey I-III).
- Displaced radial head fractures without relevant comminution (Mason II).

The available up-to-date literature is limited to individual case reports and case series with good clinical results [23–30]. The largest case series was published by Michels et al. in 2007, who performed arthroscopic osteosynthesis in 14 patients with a Mason II fracture [28]. After an average of 5.5 years, the patients had a mean Broberg/Morrey score of 97.6 points with 11 excellent and 3 good results [28].

12.3 Operating Principle/Instruments

After arthroscopically assisted anatomical reduction, the fracture can be temporarily fixed with the help of Kirschner wires before the definitive osteosynthesis is done with cannulated screws. The use of self-drilling and self-tapping screws is preferred to reduce the number of surgical steps and manipulations.

To safely avoid neurovascular complications, shear fractures of the capitulum and fractures of the coronoid are stabilized with screws from posterior to anterior. In addition to that, the iatrogenic cartilage damage can be minimized in shear fractures of the distal humerus. Ideally, at least two screws are placed to ensure adequate rotational stability. In the case of smaller fragments, adequate osteosynthesis is usually achieved with a partially threaded screw through appropriate fixation of the fragment.

The following instruments are required for arthroscopically assisted fracture treatment:

- Vacuum mattresses or the corresponding padded supports for lateral decubitus positioning of the patient.
- London-Ontario arm holder for the operated arm.
- Tourniquet cuff (optional).
- Sterile skin markers.
- Sterile 20 mL syringe and puncture cannula (for joint insufflation).
- Disposable scalpel (No. 11).
- Inflow cannula.
- Standard 4 mm arthroscope with 30-degree optic with trocar, trocar sleeve, and light source.
- Switching stick.
- Hooks.
- Arthroscopic shaver (e.g., 3.5 mm).
- Curved and straight curettes.
- Diathermy.
- Arthroscopic grasping forceps.
- Dentist hooks.
- Medium-sized, pointed, and blunt reduction clamps.
- If necessary drill guiding device (e.g., A-2096, Medartis, Fig. 12.3d).
- Tip-to-tip navigation if necessary (Brainlab) for coronoid and capitulum fractures.
- K-wires (diameter 0.8 mm and 1.1 mm).
- Cannulated drill bit (e.g., A-3736, A-3836, from Medartis) with protection sleeve.
- Cannulated, self-tapping, headless compression screws (e.g., CCS, Medartis, diameter 2.2 mm and 3.0 mm, length up to 40 mm; Biotech, diameter 1.7 mm).
- If necessary, CleverHook (Mitek).
- FiberWire 2-0 (Arthrex) and Suture Passer (Arthrex) for lasso loop refixation of the coronoid.
- C-arm.

- Sutures (e.g., 3/0, non-absorbable, monofilament) for closing the portals.

12.4 Preparation for Surgery

- History and clinical examination.
- Mechanism of trauma documentation.
- Previous operations (anterior transposition of the ulnar nerve?).
- Skin and soft tissue condition (open wounds, swelling/hematoma, preexisting scar).
- Stability test under anesthesia (medial/lateral instability, posterolateral/posteromedial rotatory instability, dislocation tendency).

Imaging

Plain radiographs of the elbow in an anteroposterior and lateral view form the basics of diagnostic imaging. A computer tomography with 3D reconstruction is carried out for operative planning. Zones of comminution or multifragmentary fractures, relevant concomitant pathologies, or involvement of the radial neck with radial head fractures can be assessed in detail using CT and are decisive for the indication or contraindication of arthroscopically assisted osteosynthesis. In addition, the CT allows precise localization and size assessment of the fragments. In this way, the screw length can be measured preoperatively and the positioning angle or the entry/exit point of the screws can be also planned.

12.5 Surgical Technique

The procedure is performed under general anesthesia with the patient lying on his/her side (lateral decubitus position). The affected upper extremity is attached to a London-Ontario arm holder in 90-degree flexion. Here, the surgeon must ensure preoperatively that the position allows a sufficient range of motion for the operated arm and, in particular, that there are no obstacles to flex the elbow. After sterile draping, a tourniquet is applied (200–250 mmHg) (optional). Relevant anatomical landmarks (tip of the olecranon, radial head, capitulum, trochlea, ulnar nerve) are drawn, and prophylactic IV antibiotics must be administered at least 20 min before the elevation of the tourniquet. This is followed by joint insufflation with 20–30 mL NaCl solution via the "soft-spot portal" and then the creation of an anterolateral irrigation portal is done. The filling of the joint is limited by the presence of hemarthrosis.

To avoid postoperative complications, it is extremely important to keep the pump pressure as low as possible (20–30 mmHg). In case of high pump pressure, the rinsing fluid can quickly distribute in the surrounding soft tissue through the joint capsule, which is often ruptured. On the one hand, increasing soft tissue swelling will make the arthroscopy more difficult; on the other hand, it can lead to postoperative compartment syndrome. The skin incisions should therefore be made somewhat larger to ensure that the arthroscopic fluid will be drained out properly through the portals.

Before treating the fracture, a diagnostic arthroscopy takes place to discover the accompanying pathologies and include them accordingly in the therapeutic approach. The C-Arm should come from the patient's foot side and should be covered by a sterile drape. In this way, X-rays can be carried out intraoperatively without hindering the surgeon.

12.5.1 Shear Fractures of the Capitulum

For arthroscopically assisted osteosynthesis of coronal shear fractures of the distal humerus, the arthroscopy begins in the posterior compartment (Figs. 12.1 and 12.2). The fracture hematoma can thus be removed, and the fracture can be visualized via the high posterolateral portal. The fracture bed is debrided via an additional posterolateral soft-spot portal with the aid of a shaver and curved curettes. Once the debridement is complete, a switch is made to the anterior compartment of the joint. An attempt can be made to reduce the fracture in a closed manner by extend-

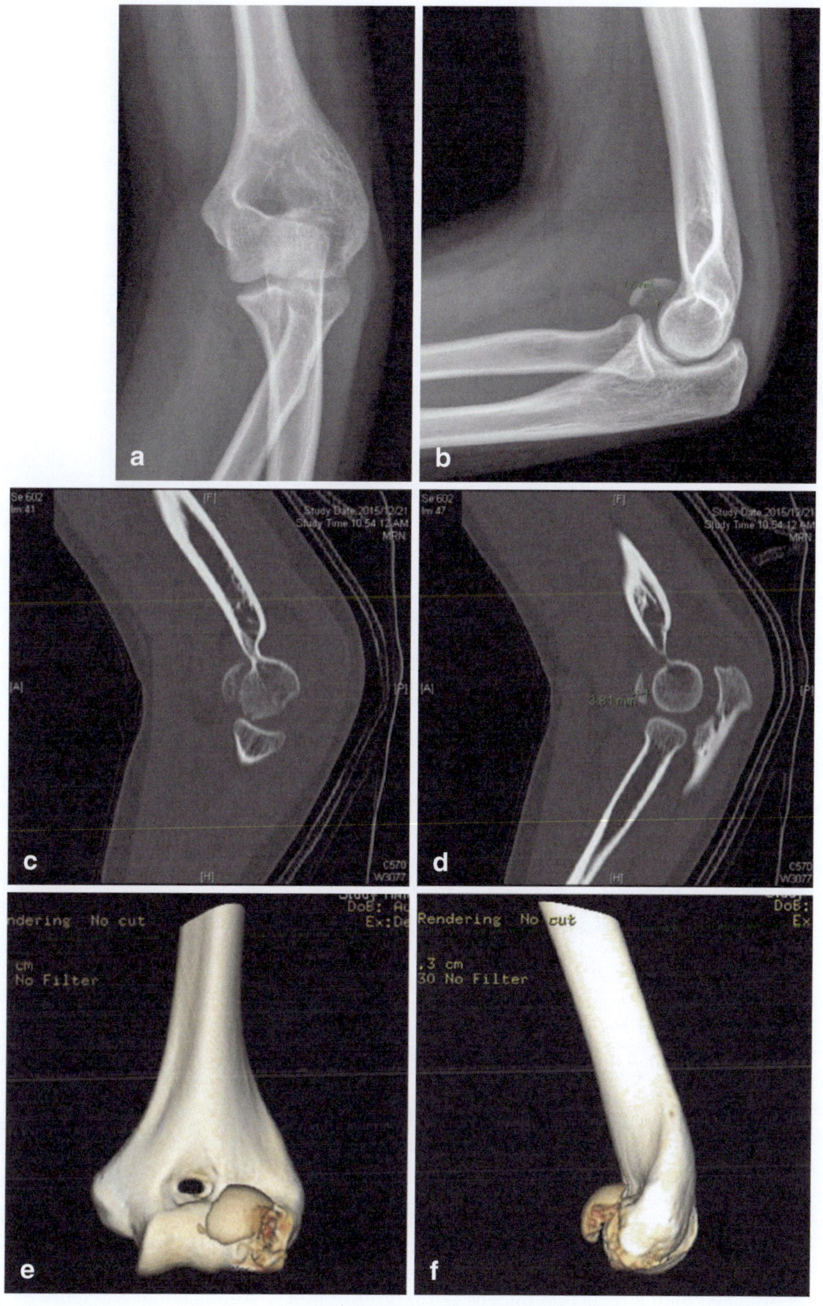

Fig. 12.1 Preoperative imaging of a 17-year-old female patient with a Dubberley IA fracture after falling on her left extended arm. (**a**, **b**) Conventional X-ray in two planes, (**c**–**f**) sagittal and 3D reconstruction with presentation of the proximally displaced, osteochondral fragment

ing the elbow in supination and under varus stress. If this does not succeed, the fragment must be reduced arthroscopically. The camera is introduced through the anteromedial portal to visualize the fracture. The switching stick can be placed proximal to the fragment via an anterolateral portal to reduce it.

The reduction can then be optimized and held with a dentist's hook or reduction forceps. The elbow is flexed at least 90 degrees to aid the reduction through a radiocapitellar compression.

In the next step, 2–3 K-wires are inserted, starting retrograde from the dorsal capitulum (depending on the size of the fragment) and inserting them

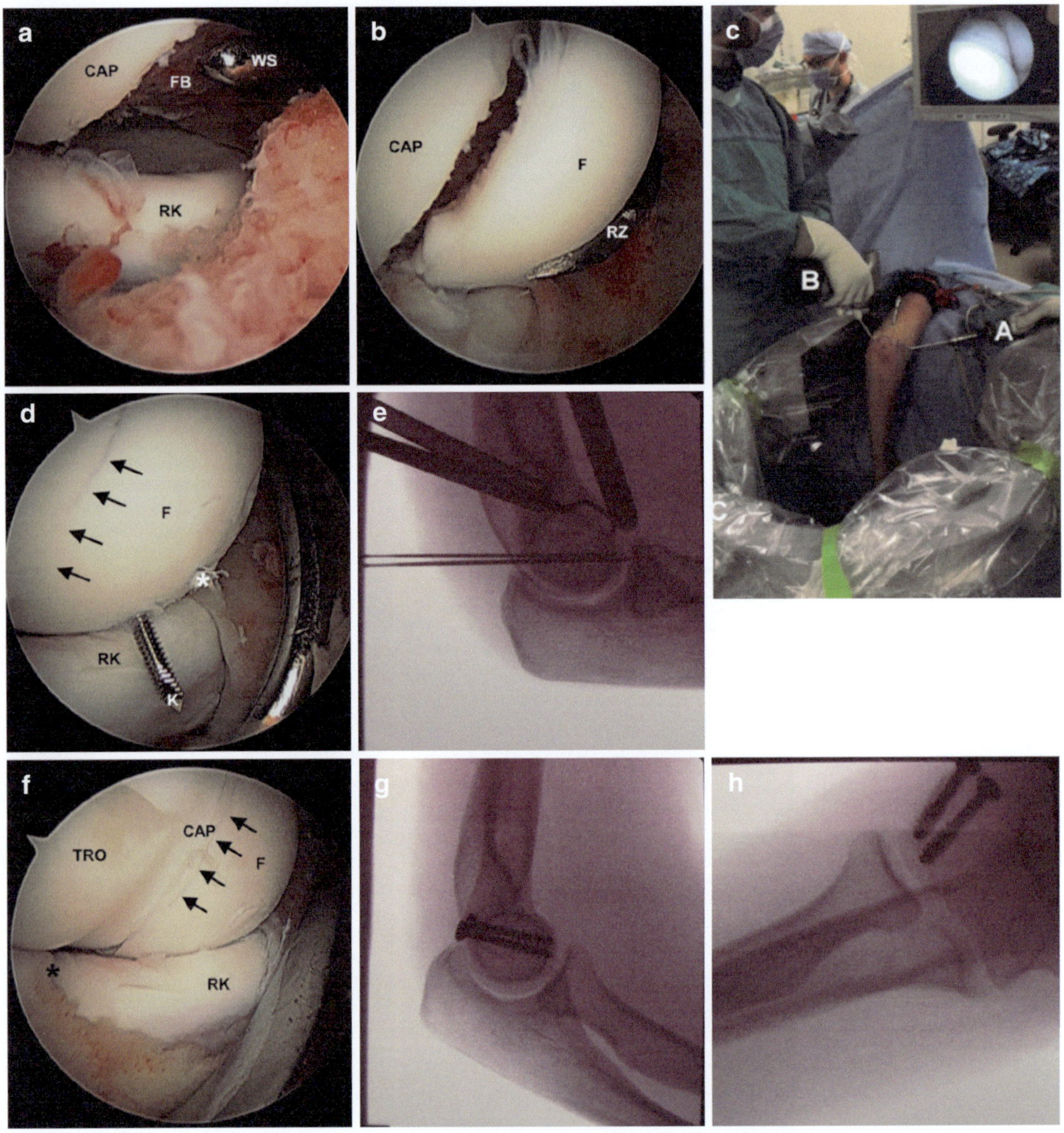

Fig. 12.2 Intraoperative findings viewed from anteromedial portal with anterolateral working portals. (**a**) After debridement of fracture bed (FB), the capitulum (CAP). The radius head (RK) is intact. (**b**) The fragment (F) is repositioned with a reduction forceps (RZ). (**c**) Insertion of the K-wires from dorsal in a retrograde manner into the reduced fragment. (**d**) The fragment (F) is anatomically reduced; the fracture gap (arrows) is now reduced. The joint is flexed so that the radial head (RK) supports the reduction. After a K-wire (K) has already been pre-drilled, a second K-wire is placed laterally parallel to it (*). (**e**) Image intensifier control in the lateral view shows the correct placement of the K-wires. (**f**) After inserting the lag screws, the K-wires were removed. The fragment (F) is still anatomically reduced; the fracture gap (arrows) can hardly be seen (* proximal radial ulnar joint). (**g**, **h**) Final image intensifier control in two planes. *A* arthroscope, *B* drill bit, *C* C-arm, *CAP* capitulum, *RK* radius head, *TRO* trochlea, *WS* switching stick

90° to the fracture line, the reduction and K-wire position should be checked using an image intensifier to avoid drilling errors or iatrogenic cartilage damage. We recommend using a guiding device (e.g., A-2096, Medartis) or tip-to-tip navigation using a 3D navigation system (e.g., Brainlab).

A pointer is positioned at the desired exit point of the wire and is shown in three dimensions in the navigation unit. The drill sleeve for drilling the K-wire and the K-wire is prepared, the surgeon can now pre-drill the K-wire in the direction of the pointer by orienting himself on the screen display. An additional radiation exposure through CT referencing is not necessary.

There is no need to use a depth gauge, since the position of the respective K-wire can be shown arthroscopically, and the screw length can be measured using its penetration depth. The cannulated, self-tapping partially threaded screws are inserted posteriorly, and the Kirschner wires are then removed. While screwing the screws, it is advisable to stabilize the reduction from the anterior side using reduction forceps, a dentist's hook, or a switching stick to avoid dislocation of the anterior fragment by the screw tip. Since the entry point of the screws generally does not communicate with the radial head in extension, the use of headless compression screws is not absolutely necessary.

The correct fracture reduction is then verified and documented arthroscopically and with the help of the image intensifier. A dorsal screw impingement must be ruled out by passively moving the elbow.

12.5.2 Coronoid Fractures

Coronoid fractures (Figs. 12.3, 12.4, 12.5, 12.6, and 12.7) can be treated arthroscopically with the aid of lag screws or—especially in the case of small fragments—with a "lasso loop technique." The fracture is visualized via an anterolateral portal, and then an anteromedial working portal is created. The fracture bed is then freed from the fracture hematoma with a shaver or curved curettes. If the fracture extends medially as in anteromedial facet fractures subtype 3 according to O'Driscoll, an open approach must be considered, as the ulnar nerve runs directly dorsal to the sublime tubercle and thus comes in the way of arthroscopic fracture reduction and osteosynthesis and could be injured.

Since the coronoid fracture is a frequent concomitant injury of a posterior elbow dislocation, additional osteochondral lesions or loose bodies must be excluded, typically in the area of the trochlear groove, the radial head, or the posterior part of the capitulum (Osborne-Cotterill lesion; [31]). In addition, the joint stability must be assessed, and depending on the findings, additional collateral ligament stabilization must be considered.

For the temporary reduction of the coronoid fragment, a medium-sized, pointed reduction forceps with a large offset is used, one end is applied to the dorsal side of the ulnar edge and the other end is applied on the fragment via the anteromedial portal. Depending on the size of the fragment, if possible two K-wires are inserted retrograde from the dorsal ulnar edge to stabilize the fracture.

Here, the use of a guide device or tip-to-tip navigation is advisable. To minimize the risk of intraarticular misalignment, the K-wire should be drilled strictly horizontally. The proximal radioulnar joint must be taken into account when drilling the lateral K-wire. An image intensifier check is rarely needed here, as the fracture reduction and the positioning of the K-wires can be assessed arthroscopically.

The very hard dorsal cortex of the ulna must be drilled with a cannulated drill in the following step before the compression screws can be inserted. The length of the screws can be measured by the depth gauge or by the depth of the K-wire or by a guide device. Due to the exposed position of the dorsal ulnar edge, we use headless compression screws, which are countersunk accordingly to avoid soft tissue irritation postoperatively. It is not always possible to place two screws, especially with small fragments. Due to the compression effect of the screw, one screw is often sufficient here.

To avoid rotation of the fragment while screwing, a second K-wire should be inserted temporarily, or the fragment should alternatively be stabilized with a dentist's hook or reduction forceps.

Alternatively, the lasso loop technique can be used for small, transverse fragments. Using tip-to-tip navigation or with the aid of a guide device, holes are drilled on the medial and lateral edges of the fracture, starting from the dorsal

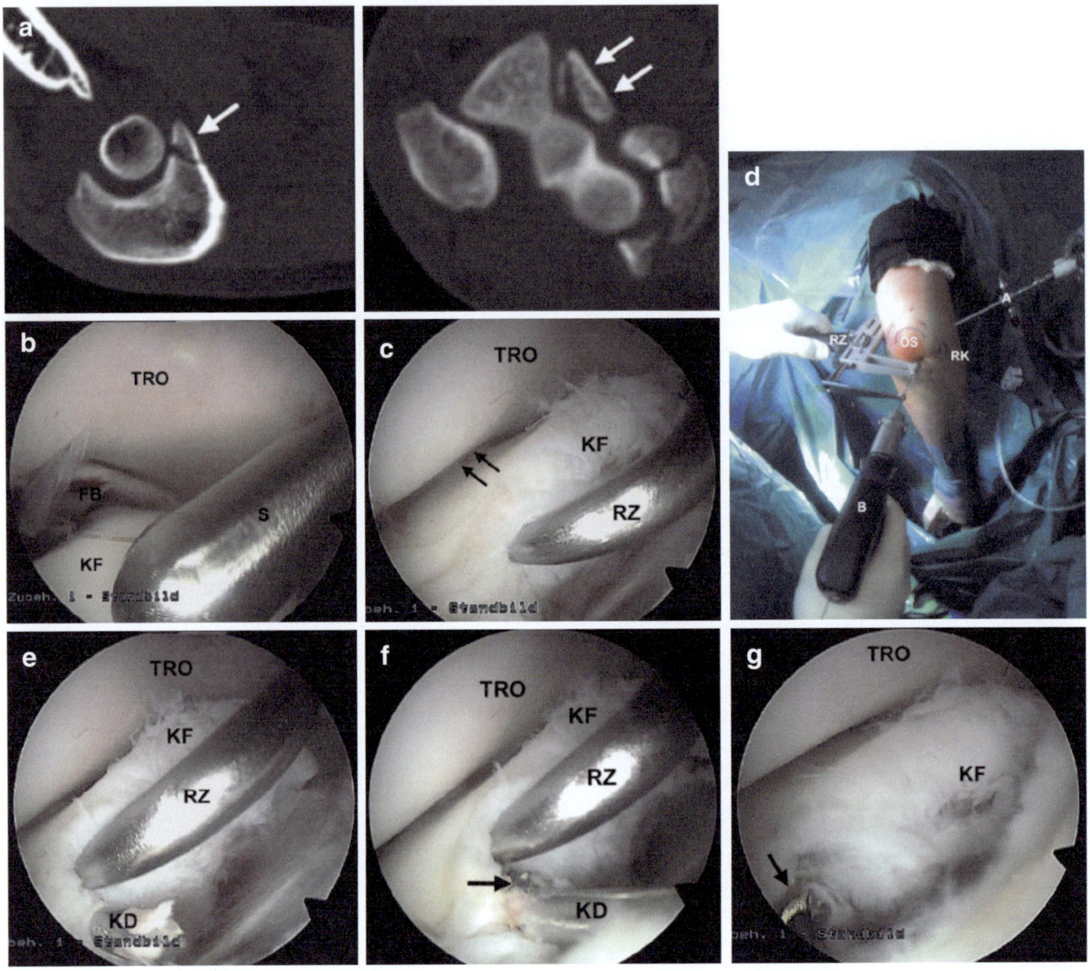

Fig. 12.3 A 30-year-old male patient with a terrible triad injury of the right elbow: preoperative imaging and intraoperative findings. (**a**) Preoperative CT showing the Regan/Morrey type II fracture (arrows) and the multifragmentary radius head fracture (Mason III). (**b**) Intraoperative findings: the arthroscope is located in the anterolateral portal. The coronoid fragment (KF) is dislocated distally. Behind it, the fracture bed (FB) with hematoma. (**c**) Reduction of the fragment (KF) with a reduction forceps (RZ) inserted through the anteromedial portal. The fracture (arrows) is anatomically reduced. (**d**) Posterior view of the elbow. The arthroscope is in the anterolateral portal. The reduction forceps (RZ) serve as a targeting device for the retrograde drilling (B) of the K-wire starting from the dorsoulnar cortex. It rests with one end on the dorsal ulnar edge and with the other through the anteromedial portal on the coronoid fragment. (**e**) Retrograde insertion of the K-wire (KD) into the lateral part of the fragment (KF). (**f**) Insertion of the cannulated compression screw (arrow) over the K-wire (KD). (**g**) Properly inserted compression screw (arrow) after removal of the K-wire. *KF* coronoid fragment, *OS* olecranon tip, *RK* radius head, *RZ* reduction forceps, *S* shaver, *TRO* trochlea

ulnar edge. A clever hook is used to enter the anteromedial portal and a FiberWire 2-0 in the form of a horizontal mattress suture is looped through the capsule adjoining the coronoid fragment. With the help of a suture passer, the respective thread ends are shuttled dorsally through the medial and lateral drill holes. The fracture can be reduced by gently pulling the thread ends alternately. If the fragment is incorrectly rotated, it can be gripped with grasping forceps and stabilized while the thread ends are tensioned. If the fracture is properly reduced, the FiberWire can be tied over the dorsal ulnar cortex to complete the osteosynthesis.

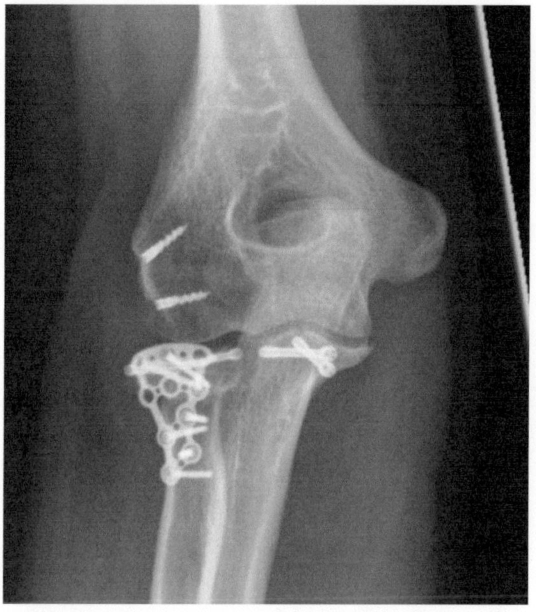

Fig. 12.4 X-ray 6 months postoperatively with consolidation of the fracture and proper implant position

12.5.3 Radial Head Fractures

Radial head fractures (Figs. 12.8, 12.9, and 12.10) are associated with a large number of cases with relevant injuries to the surrounding ligamentous structures [16]. It is therefore essential to carefully check the joint stability as part of the diagnostic arthroscopy and, if necessary, to repair the medial and/or lateral collateral ligament after fixing the fracture. In the posterior part of the joint, care must be taken to ensure that there are no loose bodies in the olecranon fossa and—as already mentioned above—in the area of the dorsal capitulum (Osborne-Cotterill lesion; [31]). If the fracture turns out to be fragmented (comminuted), which can be diagnosed in the preoperative images, then switching to an open approach must be considered at an early stage.

The fragments of the radial head, which are usually located anteriorly, can only be seen

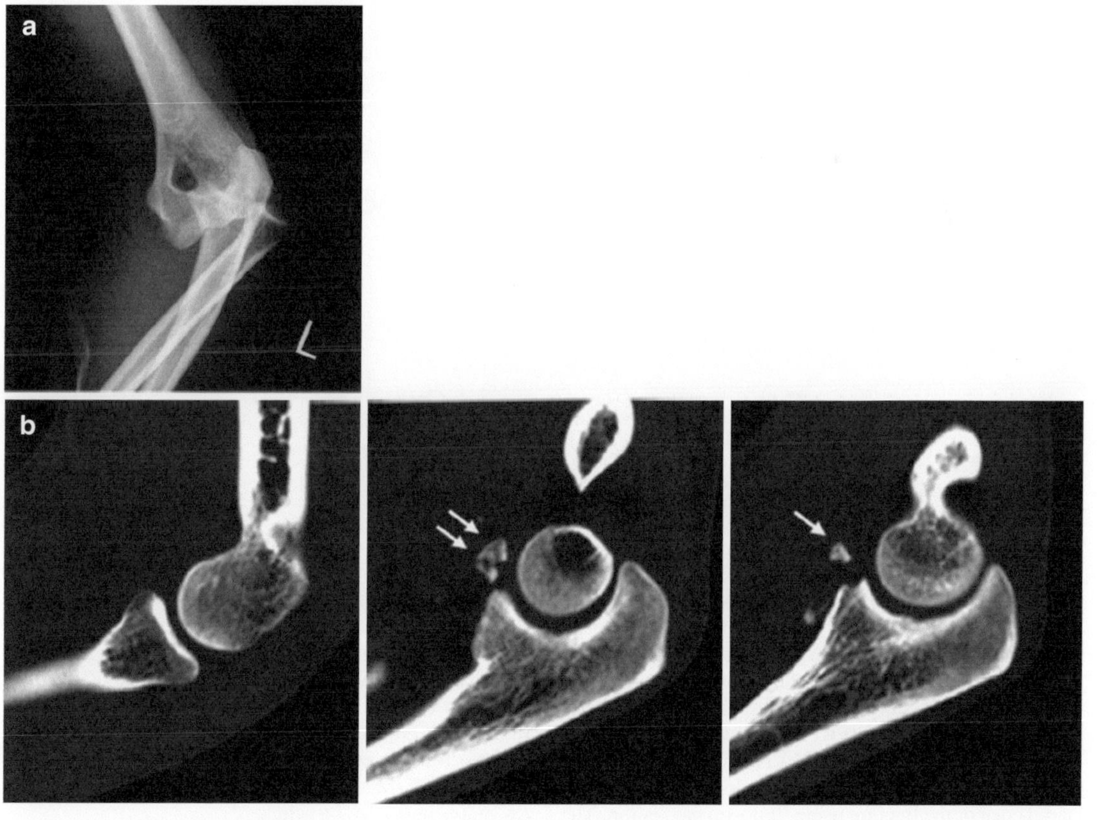

Fig. 12.5 A 30-year-old female patient presented with a coronoid fracture after left elbow dislocation. (**a**) Initial X-ray in the dislocated state. (**b**) Sagittal images after reduction with an intact radial head and a Regan/Morrey type II fracture of the coronoid

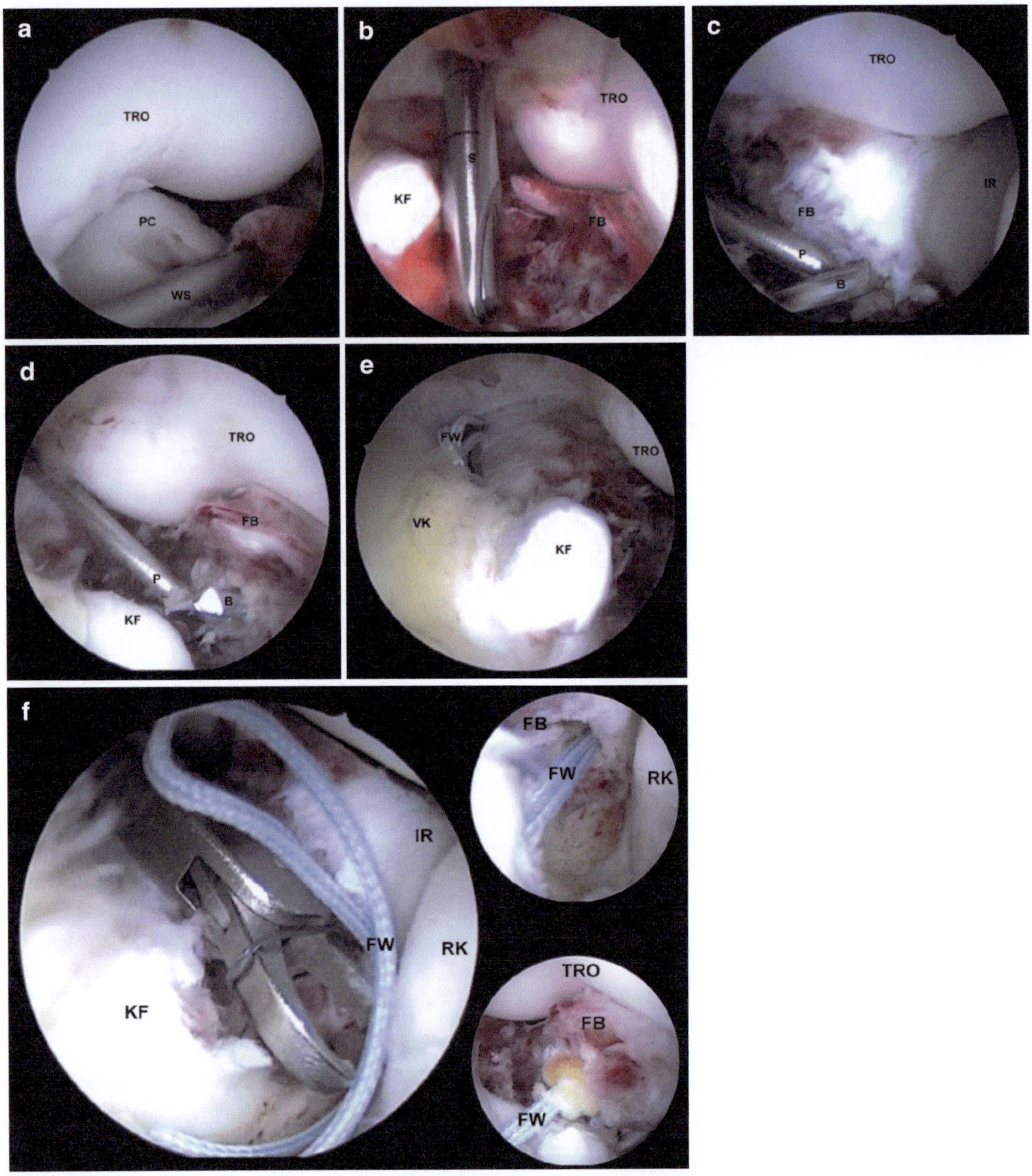

Fig. 12.6 Coronoid fixation using the lasso loop technique. (**a**) Posterolateral view through the high posterolateral portal. A switching stick (WS) was inserted through the posterolateral soft-spot portal, which can easily be pushed forward medially. The joint is clearly gaping and unstable both medially and posterolaterally. (**b**) Viewing the anterior joint compartment through an anterolateral portal. The fracture bed (FB) is cleaned with the shaver (S). The coronoid fragment (KF) is displaced anteriorly. (**c**) Creation of a retrograde 2.6 mm drill hole (B) on the lateral edge of the fracture using tip-to-tip navigation. The pointer (P) lies in the anterolateral portal. (**d**) Creation of a drill hole (B) on the medial edge of the fracture (equivalent to c). (**e**) Slinging the ventral capsule (VK) using the CleverHook. This is inserted anterolaterally and is loaded with a FiberWire (FW). (**f**) Left: Using grasping forceps, the FiberWire (FW) is placed in the eyelet of a suture passer and thus directed dorsally through the drill holes. Right: The FiberWire at the lateral (above) and medial (below) fracture edge. *FB* fracture bed, *IR* radial notch, *KF* coronoid fragment, *P* pointer, *PC* coronoid process, *RK* radius head, *TRO* trochlea

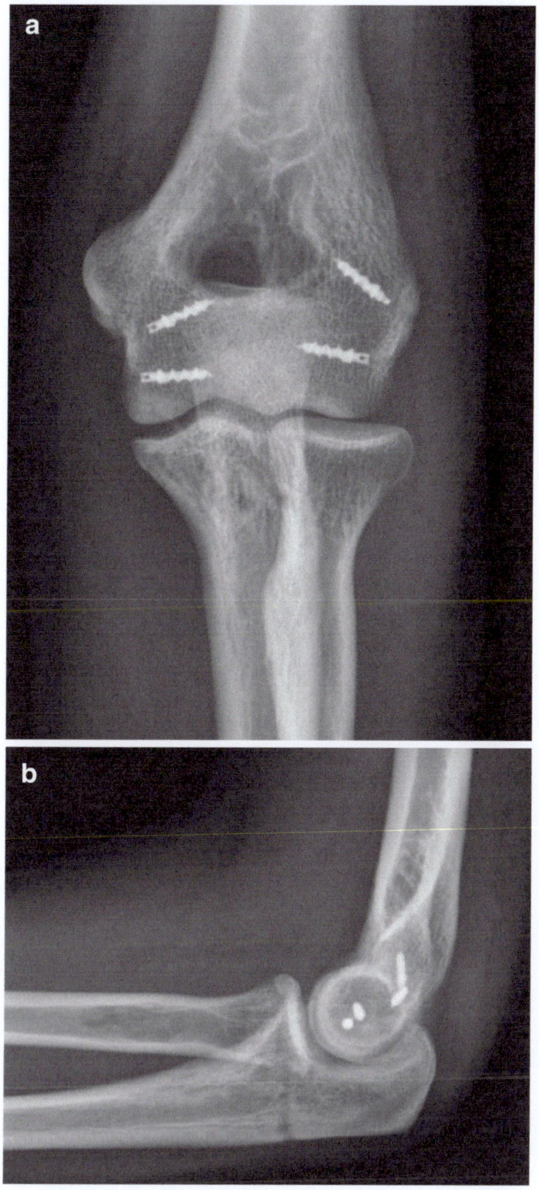

Fig. 12.7 X-ray control 2 weeks postoperatively. Correct articulation and implant position (**a**). The ulnar drill holes are still visible in the lateral projection (b)

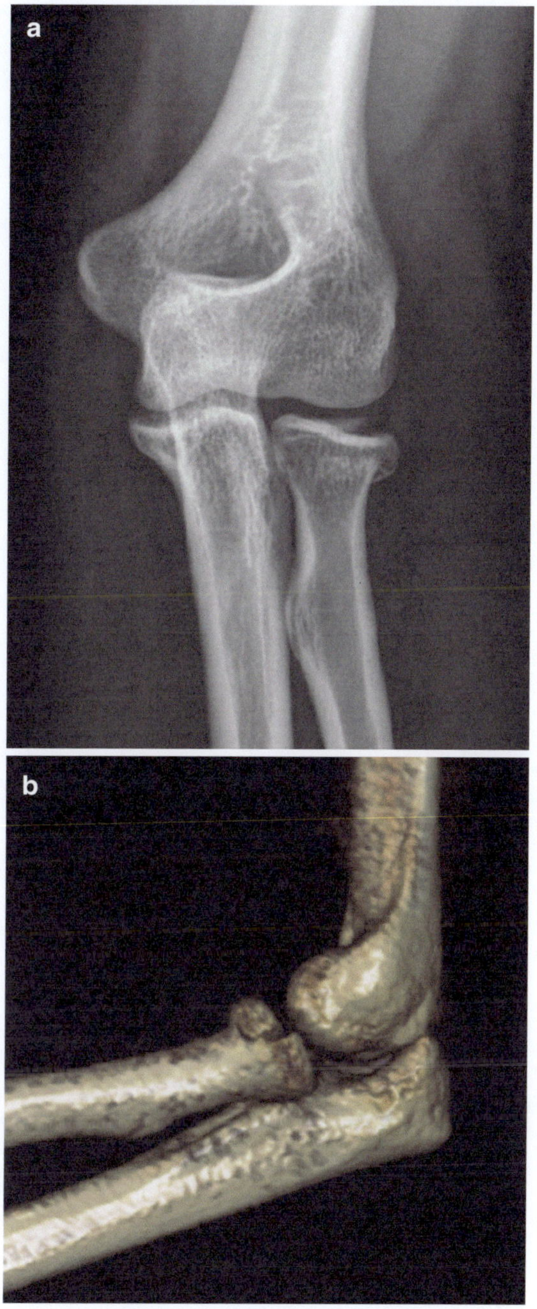

Fig. 12.8 (**a**, **b**) Preoperative X-ray and 3D CT reconstruction of a Mason type II fracture of left elbow

through the high posterolateral and the posterolateral soft-spot portal, but better exposure is usually achieved through the anterior joint compartment. The arthroscope is introduced through an anteromedial portal and the fracture hematoma is carefully removed with a shaver or curette through the anterolateral portal to expose the fracture.

The fragments can be reduced via the anterolateral portal with a dentist's hook and the reduction is held temporarily with pointed reduction forceps; two K-wires are then introduced via the posterolateral portal. The forearm is rotated so

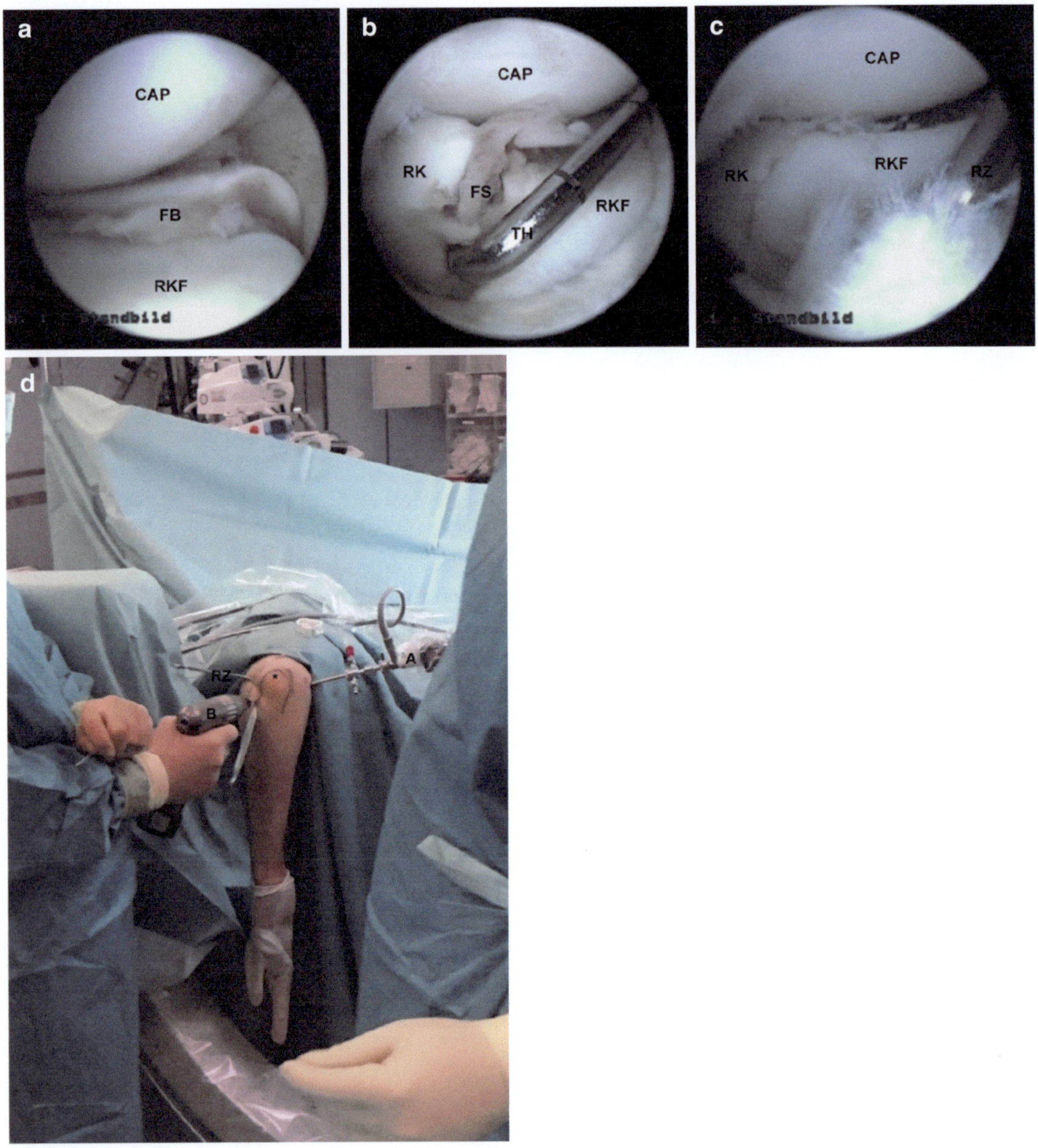

Fig. 12.9 Intraoperative findings. (**a**) Anterior view via an anteromedial portal. The radial head fragment (RKF) is dislocated distally. (**b**) The fracture gap (FS) is cleaned and palpated with a hook (TH) via the anterolateral portal. (**c**) After debridement of the fracture gap, the fragment (RKF) is anatomically reduced and temporarily fixed with reduction forceps (RZ). (**d**) The two ends of the reduction forceps (RZ) grasp the radial head via the anterolateral and the posterolateral portal. The arthroscope is located in the anteromedial portal. A 0.8 mm K-wire is pre-drilled through the posterolateral portal (B), and a cannulated, headless compression screw is inserted over it. *CAP* capitulum, *FB* fracture bed, *RK* radius head, *RKF* radius head fragment

that the fracture gap is perpendicular to the direction of drilling. The fracture reduction is checked arthroscopically, and the screw length is determined by the penetration depth of the K-wires. Since the screws often have to be placed outside the "safe zone," headless compression screws should be used, which can be introduced safely below the cartilage level at both ends. To ensure this, the respective screw should be selected about 4 mm shorter than measured to rule out protrusion of the screw with corresponding radioulnar impingement. In the case of small frag-

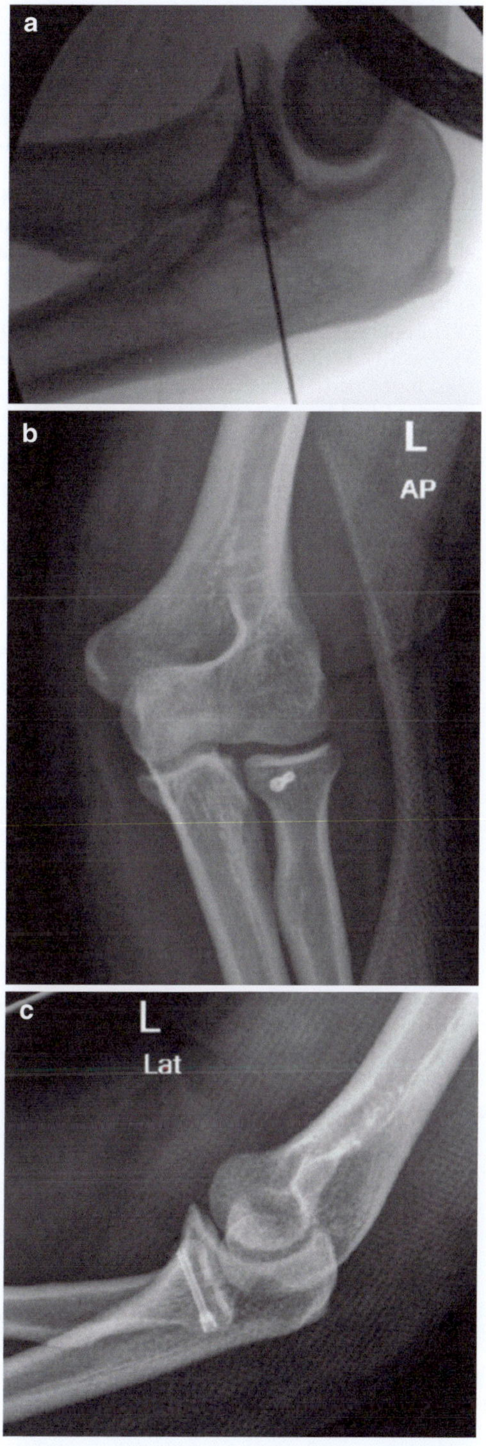

Fig. 12.10 Intra- and postoperative imaging. (**a**) Intraoperative image intensifier control of the inserted K-wire. (**b**, **c**) Postoperative X-ray in two planes. The fracture is anatomically reduced with the compression screw in place

ments, equivalent to coronoid fractures, it may be sufficient to place only one compression screw to achieve sufficient rotational stability by interdigitation of the fragments. Finally, the correct screw position and adequate fracture reduction should be verified arthroscopically and by using an image intensifier. With complete pronation and supination, radioulnar impingement by screws or joint steps must be excluded.

12.6 Postoperative Measures

Immediately after the operation, the operated arm is wrapped in an elastocompressive bandage, and antiswelling measures (cooling and elevation) are applied. If there was a relevant instability intraoperatively, a hinged elbow orthosis (e.g., Donjoy X-Act ROM Elbow, from DJO Global or Epico ROM, from medi) can be applied to protect the repaired ligaments after the operation. The pain therapy is carried out with a nonsteroidal anti-inflammatory drug (e.g., ibuprofen or diclofenac) and, if necessary, with a low-potency opioid according to the WHO grading scheme. Manual lymph drainage and physiotherapy take place from the first postoperative day. If a drainage has been inserted, it is removed on the second postoperative day.

Aftercare

The follow-up treatment is carried out depending on the injury pattern. Capitulum fractures are usually treated freely regarding the ROM. In the case of radial head and coronoid fractures, a 6-week treatment with an elbow orthosis is usually carried out with a 20-degree extension limit for 4 weeks to protect the collateral ligaments. Rotational movements should only be performed in 90-degree flexion for 6 weeks to avoid posterolateral/posteromedial rotatory forces. After 6 weeks, radiological follow-up by plain radiography is done, and careful loading is started.

Tips and Tricks

- The arthroscopic pump pressure should be as low as possible (approx. 20 mmHg) and the skin incisions should be sufficiently large to allow extravasation of arthroscopic fluids through them and to avoid postoperative complications due to soft tissue swelling (e.g., compartment syndrome).

- Accompanying pathologies must be searched for in a targeted manner, and, in particular, ligamentous joint instability must be recognized and treated additionally.
- Guiding devices or tip-to-tip navigation are helpful when creating the drill holes.
- The use of self-drilling and self-tapping screws reduces the work steps and thus the risk of displacement of the fracture reduction before completion of the osteosynthesis.
- The respective screw length can often be determined preoperatively by CT.
- In small fragments, a singular compression screw in the center of the fragment is sufficient to ensure adequate rotational stability by interlocking the fragments.
- The image intensifier is inserted under the sterile cover from the patient's foot side. Thereby, intraoperative imaging of the elbow can be performed without restricting the surgeon.

References

1. Resnick D, Kang HS. Internal derangements of joints. Philadelphia, PA: WB Saunders; 1997.
2. Doornberg JN, van Duijn PJ, Linzel D, et al. Surgical treatment of intra-articular fractures of the distal part of the humerus. Functional outcome after twelve to thirty years. J Bone Joint Surg Am. 2007;89(7):1524–32. https://doi.org/10.2106/JBJS.F.00369.
3. Guitton TG, Zurakowski D, van Dijk NC, Ring D. Incidence and risk factors for the development of radiographic arthrosis after traumatic elbow injuries. J Hand Surg. 2010;35(12):1976–80. https://doi.org/10.1016/j.jhsa.2010.08.010.
4. Herbertsson P, Josefsson PO, Hasserius R, et al. Uncomplicated Mason type-II and III fractures of the radial head and neck in adults. A long-term follow-up study. J Bone Joint Surg Am. 2004;86-A(3):569–74.
5. Dubberley JH, Faber KJ, Macdermid JC, Patterson SD, King GJ. Outcome after open reduction and internal fixation of capitellar and trochlear fractures. J Bone Joint Surg Am. 2006;88(1):46–54. https://doi.org/10.2106/JBJS.D.02954.
6. Aitken SA, Jenkins PJ, Rymaszewski L. Revisiting the 'bag of bones': functional outcome after the conservative management of a fracture of the distal humerus. J Bone Joint Surg. 2015;97-B(8):1132–8. https://doi.org/10.1302/0301-620X.97B8.35410.
7. Nauth A, McKee MD, Ristevski B, Hall J, Schemitsch EH. Distal humeral fractures in adults. J Bone Joint Surg Am. 2011;93(7):686–700. https://doi.org/10.2106/JBJS.J.00845.
8. Ries C, Wegmann K, Hackl M, Burkhart JK, Müller PL. Secondary total elbow arthroplasty after distal humeral fracture. Obere Extremität. 2014;9(3):156–62. https://doi.org/10.1007/s11678-014-0268-y.
9. O'Driscoll SW, Jupiter JB, Cohen MS, Ring D, McKee MD. Difficult elbow fractures: pearls and pitfalls. Instr Course Lect. 2003;52:113–34.
10. Hartzler RU, Llusa-Perez M, Steinmann SP, Morrey BF, Sanchez-Sotelo J. Transverse coronoid fracture: when does it have to be fixed? Clin Orthop Relat Res. 2014;472(7):2068–74. https://doi.org/10.1007/s11999-014-3477-1.
11. Schneeberger AG, Sadowski MM, Jacob HA. Coronoid process and radial head as posterolateral rotatory stabilizers of the elbow. J Bone Joint Surg Am. 2004;86-A(5):975–82.
12. Regan W, Morrey B. Fractures of the coronoid process of the ulna. J Bone Joint Surg Am. 1989;71(9):1348–54.
13. Johnston GW. A follow-up of one hundred cases of fracture of the head of the radius with a review of the literature. Ulster Med J. 1962;31:51–6.
14. Kaas L, van Riet RP, Vroemen JP, Eygendaal D. The epidemiology of radial head fractures. J Shoulder Elbow Surg/Am Shoulder Elbow Surg. 2010;19(4):520–3. https://doi.org/10.1016/j.jse.2009.10.015.
15. Fitzpatrick MJ, Diltz M, McGarry MH, Lee TQ. A new fracture model for "terrible triad" injuries of the elbow: influence of forearm rotation on injury patterns. J Orthop Trauma. 2012;26(10):591–6. https://doi.org/10.1097/BOT.0b013e31824135af.
16. Itamura J, Roidis N, Mirzayan R, Vaishnav S, Learch T, Shean C. Radial head fractures: MRI evaluation of associated injuries. J Shoulder Elbow Surg/Am Shoulder Elbow Surg. 2005;14(4):421–4. https://doi.org/10.1016/j.jse.2004.11.003.
17. McGinley JC, Gold G, Cheung E, Yao J. MRI detection of forearm soft tissue injuries with radial head fractures. Hand. 2014;9(1):87–92. https://doi.org/10.1007/s11552-013-9561-2.
18. Trousdale RT, Amadio PC, Cooney WP, Morrey BF. Radio-ulnar dissociation. A review of twenty cases. J Bone Joint Surg Am. 1992;10:1486–97.
19. Burkhart KJ, Franke S, Wegmann K, et al. Mason I fracture – a simple injury? Unfallchirurg. 2015;118(1):9–17. https://doi.org/10.1007/s00113-013-2532-9.
20. Beingessner DM, Dunning CE, Gordon KD, Johnson JA, King GJ. The effect of radial head excision and arthroplasty on elbow kinematics and stability. J Bone Joint Surg Am. 2004;86-A(8):1730–9.

21. Mehdian H, McKee MD. Fractures of capitellum and trochlea. Orthop Clin North Am. 2000;31(1):115–27.
22. Shukla DR, Pillai G, McAnany S, Hausman M, Parsons BO. Heterotopic ossification formation after fracture-dislocations of the elbow. J Shoulder Elbow Surg/Am Shoulder Elbow Surg. 2015;24(3):333–8. https://doi.org/10.1016/j.jse.2014.11.037.
23. Adams JE, Merten SM, Steinmann SP. Arthroscopic-assisted treatment of coronoid fractures. Arthroscopy. 2007;23(10):1060–5. https://doi.org/10.1016/j.arthro.2007.05.017.
24. Fink Barnes LA, Parsons BO, Hausman M. Arthroscopic management of elbow fractures. Hand Clin. 2015;31(4):651–61. https://doi.org/10.1016/j.hcl.2015.06.011.
25. Hardy P, Menguy F, Guillot S. Arthroscopic treatment of capitellum fracture of the humerus. Arthroscopy. 2002;18(4):422–6.
26. Hausman MR, Klug RA, Qureshi S, Goldstein R, Parsons BO. Arthroscopically assisted coronoid fracture fixation: a preliminary report. Clin Orthop Relat Res. 2008;466(12):3147–52. https://doi.org/10.1007/s11999-008-0502-2.
27. Kuriyama K, Kawanishi Y, Yamamoto K. Arthroscopic-assisted reduction and percutaneous fixation for coronal shear fractures of the distal humerus: report of two cases. J Hand Surg. 2010;35(9):1506–9. https://doi.org/10.1016/j.jhsa.2010.05.021.
28. Michels F, Pouliart N, Handelberg F. Arthroscopic management of Mason type 2 radial head fractures. Knee Surg Sports Traumatol Arthrosc. 2007;15(10):1244–50. https://doi.org/10.1007/s00167-007-0378-9.
29. Mitani M, Nabeshima Y, Ozaki A, et al. Arthroscopic reduction and percutaneous cannulated screw fixation of a capitellar fracture of the humerus: a case report. J Shoulder Elbow Surg/Am Shoulder Elbow Surg. 2009;18(2):e6–9. https://doi.org/10.1016/j.jse.2008.07.007.
30. Rolla PR, Surace MF, Bini A, Pilato G. Arthroscopic treatment of fractures of the radial head. Arthroscopy. 2006;22(2):233.e1–6. https://doi.org/10.1016/j.arthro.2005.10.003.
31. Osborne G, Cotterill P. Recurrent dislocation of the elbow. J Bone Joint Surg Br. 1966;48(2):340–6.

Complications After Elbow Arthroscopy

13

Marco M. Schneider, Boris Hollinger, Rainer Nietschke, and Klaus J. Burkhart

Contents

M. M. Schneider (✉)
Praxisklinik Orthopädie Aachen, Aachen, Germany
e-mail: marco.schneider@orthopia.com

B. Hollinger
Sektion Gelenk- und Extremitätenchirurgie, Uniklinik RWTH Aachen, Aachen, Germany

R. Nietschke
University Witten/Herdecke, Witten, Germany
e-mail: nietschke@orthio.de

K. J. Burkhart
Diakonie Klinikum, Stuttgart, Germany

13.1 Introduction

Over the past decade, understanding of the anatomy and functions of the elbow joint has grown significantly. Together with technical achievements and further development of arthroscopy, the arthroscopy of the elbow has become a frequently used surgical procedure.

As a result of the development of arthroscopic procedures, indications of elbow arthroscopy have been extended, and it is now considered as an integral part of surgical therapy of the elbow joint. The arthroscopy of the elbow joint is used, among other treatment modalities, for removal of symptomatic

A. B. Imhoff, A. Lenich (eds.), *Elbow Arthroscopy and Minimal Invasive Surgery*,
https://doi.org/10.1007/978-3-031-75611-5_13

loose bodies and troublesome plicae and for osteochondral defects, septic arthritis, arthrofibrosis, epicondylopathies, osteoarthrosis, and fractures.

By expanding the indications beyond diagnostic arthroscopy, knowledge and handling of postoperative complications have also been improved [1, 2].

Elbow arthroscopy tends to be a low-risk procedure. However, due to the anatomy of the elbow joint with little subcutaneous fatty tissue and therefore little soft tissue cover, as well as the close positional relationships to important nerve structures, arthroscopy can cause serious complications. The working groups of Savoie, Kelly, and Nelson described complications with incidences of 3%, 11.8%, and 13.7% in 465, 473, and 417 elbow arthroscopies [3–5].

The high variance is best explained by Kelly at the time of the arthroscopy (1980–1998) and Nelson by the partially performed steroid infiltration at the end of the operations, which caused a significantly higher infection rate ([3, 4]). In an evaluation of a total of 6268 elbow arthroscopies, the reoperation rate was 2.2%, of which infections accounted for 0.26%, elbow stiffness was up to 0.63%, and nerve injuries accounted for 1.26% [6]. A study by Jost et al. examined the complication rate after the first 100 elbow arthroscopies by a single surgeon, which was 5% [7]. The surgeon's expertise has a significant influence on the postoperative result, and that is why a gradual approach to complex indications is recommended [8].

In addition to precise knowledge of the anatomy, a number of other factors have a significant influence on avoiding complications: the experience of the surgeon, the positioning of the patient, the location and size of the arthroscopic portals, the surgical technique, and, last but not least, the individual patient factors that can significantly influence the rate of complications. These individual influencing factors include obesity, which is associated with an increased risk of infections, nerve injuries, arthrofibrosis, and internal complications [9]. In this chapter, we will describe the complications after elbow arthroscopy and strategies to avoid them, although according to our experience, the complications after elbow arthroscopy rarely occur and can be avoided with appropriate knowledge and training.

13.2 Infection and Wound Healing Disorders

Infection is one of the most common complications after elbow arthroscopy. The incidence is between 0 and 8.9% [3, 4, 6, 10]. The elbow joint is just under the skin. Compared to other joints in the body, the soft tissue layer is thin, and the subcutaneous fat tissue is sparse. The anatomy makes the joint sensitive to external influences, including pathogens on the body surface, which can lead to prolonged wound healing with persistent secretion, fistula formation, abscesses, or intra-articular infections. A distinction should be made between superficial wound healing disorders and joint infections.

13.2.1 Preoperative Antibiotic Prophylaxis

The topic of preoperative antibiotic prophylaxis (PAP) is a controversial issue. A study by Bert et al., which shows a clear selection and performance bias, showed that the administration of an antibiotic before knee arthroscopy did not cause any difference in the postoperative infection rate (0.15% with and 0.16% without antibiotics; [11]). In a 2010 survey by Müler-Rath, 62% of the surgeons questioned stated that they administer antibiotic prophylaxis before an outpatient knee arthroscopy [12]. Kurzweil also recommends antibiotics before arthroscopy. A general recommendation of the PAP cannot be made due to the lack of evidence [13]. Rather, an individual assessment of the need should be made. The decision-making should include the risks and consequences of antibiotic therapy (allergic reactions, antibiotic resistance, colitis, etc.), previous illnesses and risk factors of the patient (diabetes mellitus, obesity, skin diseases, immunosuppression, nicotine abuse, circulatory disorders), and surgical intervention (operation time, introduction of foreign material, technical effort, change to open surgery) [12–15]. If preoperative antibiotic prophylaxis is desired, first- and second-generation cephalosporins or clindamycin is recommended in the case of intolerance to cephalosporins or penicillins [15].

Despite the lack of evidence from PAP for arthroscopies, our recommendation is also a preoperative antibiotic prophylaxis as a "single shot." The added value of repeated antibiotic prophylaxis compared to a preoperative single shot, which should ideally be administered approx. 30–59 min before the start of the operation, has not been proven and, on the contrary, can even lead to increased complications [15].

13.2.2 Superficial Wound Healing Disorders

Superficial wound problems, which include persistent wound secretion and superficial infections, are described in the literature with an incidence of approx. 7% [3, 4]. Superficial wound infections are usually characterized by redness and increased sensitivity to pain in the area of the arthroscopic portals. Depending on the clinical findings and additional symptoms, additional therapeutic measures should be considered on an individual basis. The general recommendation of prophylactic antibiotic therapy in the case of persistent wound secretion without signs of inflammation does not exist if there is no evidence, even if some authors use an oral antibiotic regimen for 7–14 days [3, 16]. Contrary to the previous practice of closing with Steri-Strips, the arthroscopic portals should be closed with skin sutures [3, 17]. Compared to the medial portals, the lateral portals are more sensitive to superficial wound problems, which can best be explained by the thinner soft tissue covering [3, 18]. In order to be able to guarantee a "watertight" closure after arthroscopy, we recommend not inserting a drain. If drainage is urgently required, we recommend diversion via an anteromedial or transtricipital portal, because there is greater soft tissue coverage there. With the procedure we have practiced without introducing a drain, no fistulas, revision-requiring hematomas, or superficial wound defects have occurred to date. The removal of hair in the operating area has no positive influence on the rate of superficial or deep wound infections [19, 20]. If hair removal is desired preoperatively, this should be done outside of the operating room and generally with what is known as "electrical shaver," similar to a beard trimmer. The use of razor blades is not recommended because they can cause microscopic skin injuries [19–21].

13.2.3 Septic Arthritis

The occurrence of joint infections after elbow arthroscopy is rare and is estimated in the literature to be up to 2.2% [4], with no postoperative infections occurring in numerous case series [16, 22, 23]. Several studies have found a direct connection between steroid infiltration at the end of the operation and an increased risk of infection, which is why such an infiltration should be avoided after arthroscopy [3, 4, 10, 24]. If joint infection is confirmed on the basis of clinical and laboratory findings and a joint puncture (microbiological), insertion of antibiotic-containing sponges is recommended. If a preoperative joint puncture has been performed, antibiotic therapy can be started immediately. If a joint puncture was not performed, the PAP should only be performed after intraoperative microbiological samples have been obtained, in order not to compromise the results. The arthroscopic irrigation with extensive debridement seems to be sufficient in septic arthritis of the elbow. The antibiotic treatment that follows the therapeutic joint irrigation or the joint puncture should initially be carried out with a broad-spectrum antibiotic, and, if the microbiological findings are obtained, it should be adjusted according to culture and sensitivity test [15, 25]. Close clinical and laboratory controls under antibiotic therapy are recommended after the operation. As a result, the indication for joint irrigation should be made to clean up the infection.

Tips

- The administration of preoperative antibiotic prophylaxis (PAP) is not evidence based, but it is recommended by us.
- When using the PAP, the patient should have a single shot. A multiple administration of antibiotics postoperatively is rarely necessary and has no added value compared to the single shot.

- Hair removal should never be done with a razor, but always with electric clipping outside of the operating room.
- Skin closure is done with stitches.
- The insertion of a drainage after elbow arthroscopy is seldom or never necessary and should be done through medial or transtricipital portals, respectively.
- Steroid infiltrations at the end of the operation are associated with a significant increase in the risk of infection.
- Superficial wound healing disorders with prolonged secretion should be treated with "wait-and-see" principle, depending on the clinical findings. If there are clear signs of infection, surgical revisions or, in the case of a purely superficial infection, short-term antibiotic therapy is recommended.
- In case of postoperative infections, arthroscopic irrigation with subsequent broad-spectrum antibiotic therapy with resistance-based adjustment is usually sufficient.

13.3 Neurological Complications

Temporary and permanent nerve injuries are frequently occurring complications after elbow arthroscopy, which are described with an incidence of up to 15% [3, 26–28] and can also occur with experienced surgeons [29]. Increasing the understanding of the anatomy of the elbow joint and improving arthroscopy technology have made it possible to reduce the incidence of neurological complications in spite of expanded indications. The case series available in the literature are mostly related to individual centers and surgeons. In a survey in the "American Society for Surgery of the Hand" (ASSH) by Desai et al., 30% of the participants stated that they had already observed nerve injuries after elbow arthroscopy. The respondents stated that regardless of the nerve affected, a total of 80% of the patients with sensory and 77% with motor deficits could not achieve complete recovery of the nerve function despite extensive therapy. As the data are relatively sparse, the number of nerve injuries could possibly be underestimated [30].

Potential injuries result on the one hand from the positional relationship of the arthroscopic portals to neural structures and on the other hand from the extension of the indication for elbow arthroscopy and the associated increased complexity of the interventions [1, 3, 31]. Rheumatoid arthritis and elbow stiffness have been identified as main risk factors, where changes in the joint capsule represent a danger in both pathologies [1, 3, 32]. In rheumatoid arthritis, the capsule is often thinned and the muscular landmarks such as the brachialis muscle are atrophied. In case of stiff elbows or arthrofibrosis, sufficient joint distension is not possible due to the reduced capsule volume, which means that the distance to endanger the neurological structures is smaller [32–34]. In contractures, if the joint can absorb fluid at all, only 6–10 mL can be injected in some cases [34]. In addition, the osteoarthritis complicates the overview in the joint, sometimes severely. In the context of arthroscopic capsulotomy, the nerve structures of the elbow joint are particularly at risk. In order to avoid neurological complications after elbow arthroscopy, the anatomy should be mastered and "safe zones" should be identified before the placement of the arthroscopic portals.

13.3.1 Radial Nerve

The radial nerve runs along the ventrolateral aspect of the elbow and divides into its deep and superficial branches at the level of the lateral epicondyle, immediately proximal to the supinator muscle. When the anterolateral portal is established, the nerve is in the immediate vicinity [27, 35–37] (Fig. 13.1).

It should be noted that the distance from the radial nerve to the capsule cannot be influenced by the position of the elbow or by joint distension. For this reason, arthroscopic arthrolysis can lead to serious injuries. Temporary affection of the radial nerve is described in the literature with an incidence of up to 7%. The symptoms are mostly regressed completely before discharge or within 6 weeks postoperatively. The use of local anesthetics, false placement of arthroscopic portals, and working with suction-inducing instruments

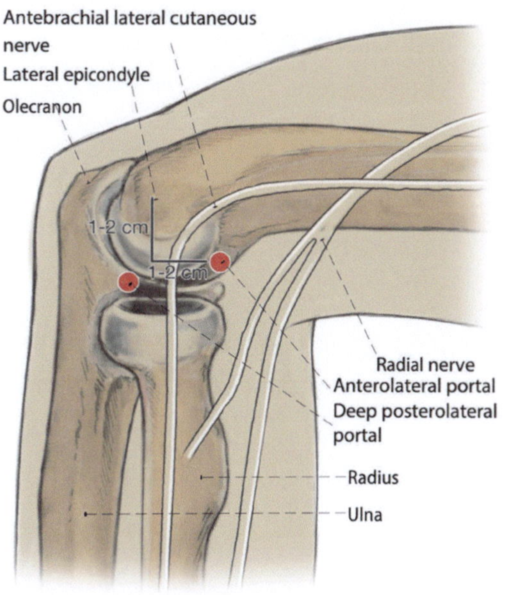

Fig. 13.1 Schematic presentation of the positional relationship between the radial nerve and portals of the arthroscopy. (Reproduced with permission from [38])

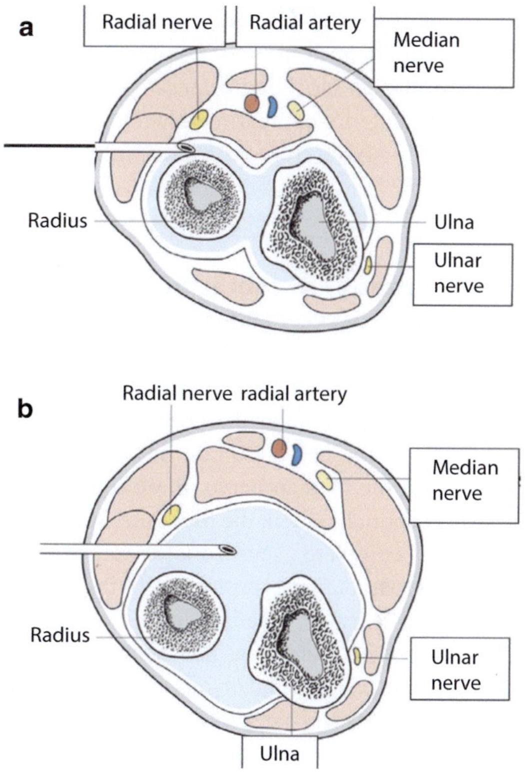

Fig. 13.2 Schematic presentation of the safety distance to the radial nerve before (**a**) and after (**b**) joint distension. (Reproduced with permission from [43])

in the area of the ventral capsule during arthrolysis have been identified as the causes of neuropathies [4, 17, 31, 39]. A complete transection of the radial nerve (and median nerve) was described by Haapaniemi in 1999, in the context of elbow arthroscopic arthrolysis of the elbow, in severe anatomical changes with chronic misalignment of the elbow and reduced capsule volume that resulted in reduction of the joint capsule distension and hence provide a very bad overview intraoperatively [40]. From our point of view, a complication rate of 7% appears to be quite high and a complete cutting of the nerve is difficult, unless the arthroscopic instruments are used in poor visibility without clear visualization of the important guide structures.

We recommend the creation of a proximal anterolateral portal in 90° flexion after joint distension with fluid, because various studies have shown increase in distances between the nerve and the portal and bone landmarks with the same intra-articular overview compared to without joint distension ([37, 41, 42]) (Fig. 13.2).

A recent and detailed work by Hackl et al. considered that the forearm rotation has no effect on the distances mentioned [41]. In case of capsule contractures, special care is required because filling of the joint before creating the first arthroscopic portal leads to an increase in the distance between the bone and the neurovascular structures, but at the same time the distance between the capsule and neurovascular structures decreases. A ventral capsulotomy should be started from the ulnar and proximal regions. Distal to the joint line, there is an increased risk of injuring the radial nerve [44]. On the ulnar side, the median nerve is better protected by the brachialis muscle. Once the layer between the capsule and muscle is shown, the capsulotomy can be completed distally and radially. The capsule can be selectively resected without damaging the muscles and nerve fibers lying on it. If the capsule is stuck with a compromised overview, a blunt dissection can first be made on the capsule before it is further excised. If the joint collapses as a result of the capsulectomy, the use of retractors is recommended in order to maintain a good overview. Under no circumstances should you work in the anterior compartment without a direct view of the shaver (or any other arthroscopic instrument).

13.3.2 Anterior Antebrachial Interosseous Nerve

The anterior antebrachial interosseous nerve represents a branch of the median nerve.

Injuries to the nerve are rare due to its distal origin from the median nerve; these injuries are described sporadically in the literature. If the dissection is complete, sensorimotor deficits are usually irreparable and permanent. In the area of the ventral capsule, there can be adhesions between the nerve and capsular tissue, which in case of arthrolysis can favor intraoperative damage [32]. The ventral capsulotomy should be carried out carefully and under vision before the elbow joint is distended.

13.3.3 Ulnar Nerve

The ulnar nerve is found on the medial side of elbow in the ulnar sulcus (groove) behind the medial epicondyle and located at risk while operating in the dorsomedial compartment and recess. If the nerve is anteriorly transferred or subluxated, it will also be at great risk when the anteromedial portal is established [45] (Fig. 13.3). Damage of the ulnar nerve is much more common than that of the other nerves and often results in surgical revision [30]. The incidence of complete dissection is about 1% [31]. In case of revision surgery with open exposure of the nerve, there are often neuromas that must be resected before reconstruction. Often, the sensomotoric deficit cannot be fully restored. Most injuries also occur here during arthroscopic arthrolysis [31, 46, 47]. Kelly et al. observed five temporary neuropathies of the ulnar nerve in a total of 473 elbow arthroscopies.

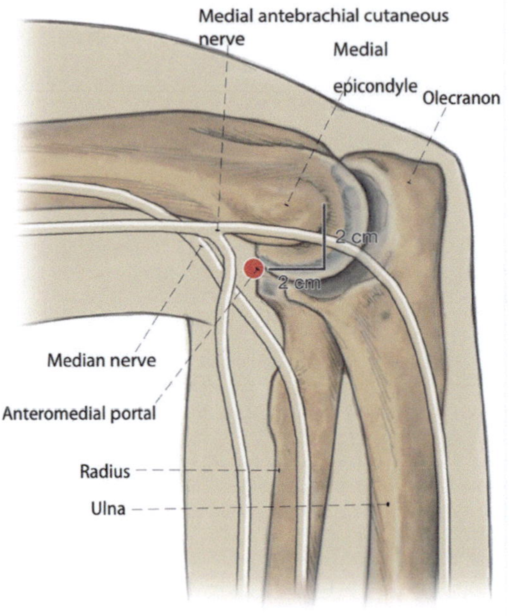

Fig. 13.3 Schematic presentation of the positional relationship between the ulnar nerve and portals of the arthroscopy. (Reproduced with permission from [38])

Three reasons are considered mainly as the causative factors for injury of the ulnar nerve:

1. Too posterior application of the anteromedial portals
2. Traction-related neuropathy after the application of "continuous passive motion therapy" with a plexus block in situ after arthroscopic arthrolysis
3. A flexion-induced neuropathy with postoperatively increased flexion also observed after arthrolysis

The complication described under number 3 had already been seen in open arthrolysis. A limited flexion-extension movement is therefore a risk factor for the development of traction-related neuropathies. In case of preoperative neuropathy of the ulnar nerve and a degree of flexion <95°, an open exposure of the nerve with retraction during arthroscopy is recommended [3, 48].

A prophylactic decompression of the ulnar nerve of about 7–8 cm will reduce the rate of irritation of the ulnar nerve from 11% to 3% [49].

The anteromedial portal therefore should not be placed too far posteriorly. Sahajpal, Blonna, and O'Driscoll provided a sensible strategy for the anteromedial portal and the associated handling of the ulnar nerve [50]. The attempt is made to feel the nerve preoperatively and to move it as far as possible anteriorly and posteriorly in order to be able to estimate the extent of the subluxation. The nerve is then fixed to the medial epicondyle if it can be palpated. The rest of the portal system is based on the palpation of the nerve (Fig. 13.4).

For orientation, palpation of the ulnar nerve can be repeated during the operation if necessary. The use of arthroscopic retractors while working with the burr is recommended, as the tissue can be sucked and damaged, and the arthroscopic exposure of the ulnar nerve intra-articularly can also avoid injuries [3, 51].

13.3.4 Remaining Neurological Structures

Remaining nerves are rarely injured, and the creation of the arthroscopic portals represents the greatest risk. In addition to the aforementioned nerves, elbow arthroscopy can injure additional nerves with exclusively sensory fibers. These include the medial antebrachial cutaneous nerve (especially the distal anteromedial portal; Fig. 13.5), the lateral antebrachial cutaneous nerve from the musculocutaneous nerve (proximal anterolateral and lateral portal; Fig. 13.1), and the posterior cutaneous antebrachial nerve from the radial nerve (proximal and distal anterolateral portal).

Tips

- Need for detailed knowledge of the anatomy.
- Preoperative marking of the bone and neural structures (especially ulnar nerve) is recommended.
- Recognition of existing preoperative risk factors (rheumatoid arthritis, elbow stiffness with reduced capsule volume, previous operations, subluxation of the ulnar nerve, obesity, etc.) and contraindications (extensive heterotopic ossifications, severe elbow stiffness, insufficient experience of the surgeon, etc.).
- Correct placement of the arthroscopic portals after previous joint distension, taking into account the recommended arm position.

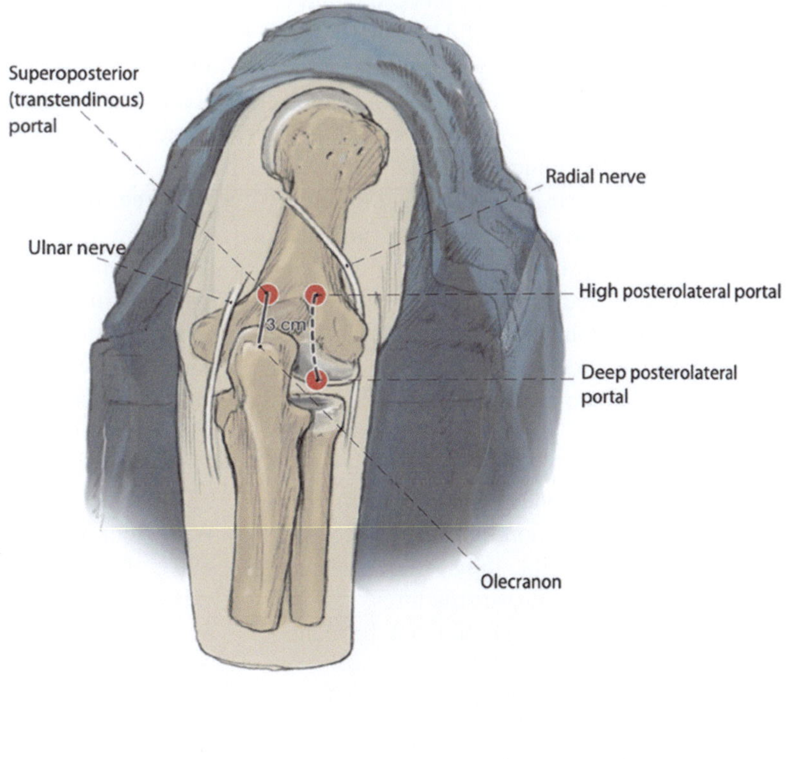

Fig. 13.4 Surgical procedure depending on the ability to palpate the ulnar nerve. (Modified according to [50]. With permission)

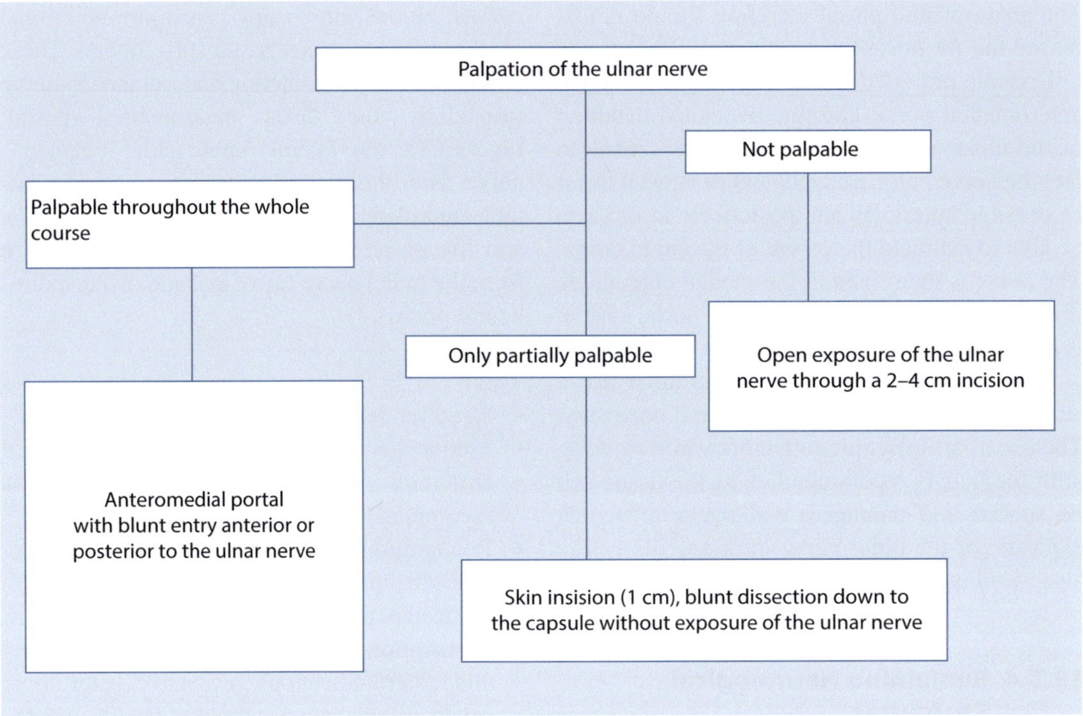

Fig. 13.5 Schematic presentation of the positional relationship between the median nerve and arthroscopic portals. (Reproduced with permission from [38])

- The proximal portal system is described as safer than the distal one.
- Only incise the skin, and then proceed bluntly. Use of a blunt trocar or careful preparation on the capsule (if the anatomy is unclear: avoid deep stab incisions).
- Forced joint distension (more than 25 mL NaCl) can lead to ruptures of the joint capsule with massive extravasation into the soft tissue. The same risk arises when using pressure pumps with a pressure setting that is too high.
- Completion of the intra-articular procedure (removal of free joint loose bodies, etc.) before capsulotomy in order to minimize the extravasation of water into the tissue.
- When using arthroscopic instruments (with and without suction), work should be carried out as close to the bone as possible in order to avoid accidental suction/injuring of the soft tissues and thus possible injury to the anterior capsule and attached nerve structures.
- The brachialis muscle should not be penetrated.
- When resecting bone parts, thin osteotomes can be used, which can minimize the risk of nerve injuries compared to the "burr."
- Increased angulation of the arthroscopic instruments can lead to compression or traction of the nerves.
- For capsulotomies, it is advisable to work close to the bone and from proximal to the joint line. If the capsulotomy is widened distally, the risk of nerve injuries increases. Arthroscopic retractors can provide a better overview in capsulotomies.
- When performing capsulotomies with unclear anatomical conditions, the arthroscopic viewing of the nerve structures from intra-articular can be useful.
- The arthroscopic instruments should always be in the field of view of the camera.
- With maximum flexion preoperatively of $<90°$, if arthrolysis is planned, due to the expected increase in mobility, open exposure of the ulnar nerve should be considered in order to avoid traction damage.

- In the case of significant subluxation and previous operations in the area of the ulnar nerve, careful dissection on the capsule or even prophylactic exposure can reduce the risk of injury.
- If necessary, open access to the elbow joint should also be mastered. If visibility is poor, you should consider converting the operation from arthroscopy to open procedure.
- The intra-articular application of a local anesthetic can mimic nerve failures, and plexus catheters lying in position can conceal neuropathies postoperatively.

13.4 Heterotopic Ossifications

Elbow stiffness can be caused by intrinsic or extrinsic causes. Heterotopic ossifications (HOs) are among the extrinsic causes. The development after elbow arthroscopy, which falls into the group of nontraumatic heterotopic ossifications, is rare, and the underlying pathological mechanism is most likely based on the release of various mediators such as prostaglandins and growth factors [52, 53]. The incidence is between 0 and 1.6%, depending on the case series [3, 4, 6]. Even if steroid infiltration is done at the end of the arthroscopy of the elbow that can reduce the risk of developing periarticular ossification, this is not recommended due to the increased risk of infection [4]. The classification preferred by the authors is based on Hastings and Graham [54].

Patients usually complain of elbow pain with involvement of the surrounding muscles and, above all, a reduction in active and passive mobility.

In the literature, there are also individual case descriptions that document HO after elbow arthroscopy. All of them were treated with open resection of the ossification with subsequent administration of indomethacin orally and, in one case, additional radiotherapy. This always showed improved mobility of the elbow joint without recurrence of the ossification [55–57].

The known risk factors for the development of periarticular ossification after operations (without previous trauma) are mainly known from hip surgery. These include the male sex, old patient age, previous occurrence of heterotopic ossifications in another location, advanced osteoarthritis, high blood pressure, obesity, and neurological concomitant diseases.

Forestier's disease (diffuse idiopathic skeletal hyperostosis, DISH) is also a risk factor and is controversial [55, 56, 58, 59]. If risk factors are present, after primary elbow arthroscopy, the 10- to 14-day use of nonsteroidal anti-inflammatory drugs can be considered, whereby the preparation of indomethacin in a dose of 50–75 mg twice a day has proven itself as an effective prophylactic method [60–63]. Another prevention method is radiotherapy, which is recommended in the literature within 72 h postoperatively with a dose of 700 cGy [58, 64–66]. In individual cases, however, the occurrence of HO was observed after a simple elbow arthroscopy without extensive capsulectomy (Fig. 13.6). The patients who tend to be at high risk are those who have undergone resection of the bony structures or in whom the capsule is detached from the bone as part of elbow arthroscopy [4, 56].

The therapeutic recommendation for extrinsic elbow stiffness induced by heterotopic ossification is usually an open resection of the ossification if there is significant restriction of mobility and after unsuccessful conservative therapy. The incision depends on the location of the ossifications [67]. The best time to operate the periarticular ossification after elbow arthroscopy has not been clearly established. Depending on the etiology of the HO, the time varies between 4 and 18 months [68, 69]. In the past, the literature advocated a "wait-and-see" attitude with manifestation of HO and resection during the course [68, 70].

In the meantime, however, an early intervention and resection of the HO were investigated [65, 69, 71, 72], whereby both strategies achieved good clinical results with a low recurrence rate.

Wert and Savoie carried out the early arthroscopic resection (within 6 weeks postoperatively) of ventral and posterior HO with subsequent radiotherapy and were also able to improve the preoperative condition. The technique

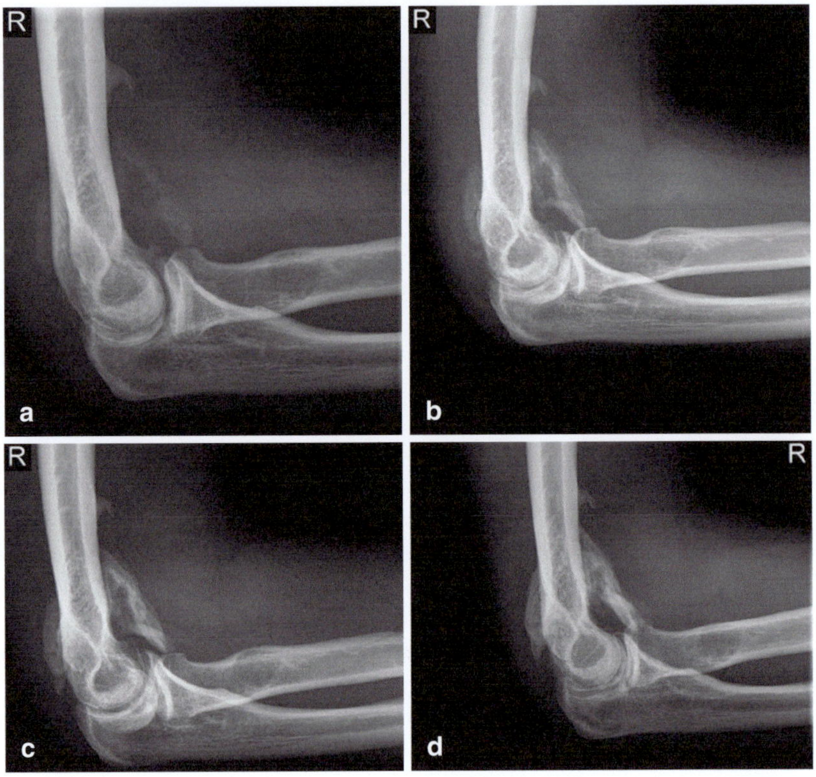

Fig. 13.6 (a–d) Development of heterotopic ossification anteriorly and posteriorly to the humerus in the lateral view after elbow arthroscopy with extensive arthrolysis, with synovectomy and capsulectomy, resection of osteophytes, and removal of free joint bodies in an elderly patient with posttraumatic arthrosis and elbow stiffness. (Courtesy of Arcus Sportklinik, Pforzheim 2018. All Rights Reserved)

described requires a high level of anatomical and arthroscopic knowledge. After detaching the capsule, exposing the ossification, and protecting neural structures with a retractor, the resection is performed with a shaver. The precautionary measures already mentioned apply here too; in particular, the brachialis muscle should be used as a reference [73, 74].

After elbow arthroscopy, the time of operation for HO should be determined individually depending on secondary diseases, extent of elbow stiffness including soft tissue shortening, and potential risk of osteoarthritis and should be based on the surgeon's skills (open vs. arthroscopic).

Tips

- Gentle resection of bone, other structures, and capsule/soft tissue.
- Adequate hemostasis and thorough rinsing of the joint to remove debris.
- For high-risk patients, postoperatively, consider prophylaxis of ossification with 50–75 mg indomethacin twice daily for approx. 2 weeks and, if necessary, radiotherapy within 72 h.
- The optimal time for removing HO has not been definitively determined but should not be delayed too much in order to avoid shortening of the soft tissue and damage to the cartilage.

13.5 Other Complications

Other rare complications including arthrofibrosis, which is most likely to occur in patients with osteochondral defects (osteoarthritis, osteochondritis dissecans, local cartilage damage, etc.), with an incidence of 0.63–3%, usually have a good response to early postoperative passive-assisted physiotherapy [3, 4, 6]. Intra-articular breakage of instruments with difficulty of removal is also reported [75].

The complex regional pain syndrome (CRPS) and postoperative hematoma formation should also be mentioned, although both complications represent general risks after surgical treatment of the upper extremity and either limit themselves or respond well to physiotherapy and pain therapy [7]. The occurrence of olecranon bursitis following elbow arthroscopy is also described with an incidence of 0.6% [76].

Complications associated with tourniquet are very rare and mainly correlate with a duration of tourniquet application. Damage at the cellular level occurs after a short time, but is almost invariably reversible without specific therapy, provided that the duration did not exceed 2 h. It is therefore recommended to use the tourniquet for a maximum of 2 h, although this recommendation cannot be justified with clear evidence [77].

References

1. Adams JE, King GJ, Steinmann SP, Cohen MS. Elbow arthroscopy: indications, techniques, outcomes, and complications. Instr Course Lect. 2015;64:215–24.
2. Bennett JM. Elbow arthroscopy: the basics. J Hand Surg Am. 2013;38(1):164–7. https://doi.org/10.1016/j.jhsa.2012.10.023.
3. Kelly EW, Morrey BF, O'Driscoll SW. Complications of elbow arthroscopy. J Bone Joint Surg Am. 2001;83-A(1):25–34.
4. Nelson GN, Wu T, Galatz LM, Yamaguchi K, Keener JD. Elbow arthroscopy: early complications and associated risk factors. J Shoulder Elb Surg. 2014;23(2):273–8. https://doi.org/10.1016/j.jse.2013.09.026.
5. Savoie FH 3rd. Complications. In: Savoie 3rd FH, Field LD, editors. Arthroscopy of the elbow. New York, NY: Churchill Livingstone; 1996.
6. Leong NL, Cohen JR, Lord E, Wang JC, McAllister DR, Petrigliano FA. Demographic trends and complication rates in arthroscopic elbow surgery. Arthroscopy. 2015;31(10):1928–32. https://doi.org/10.1016/j.arthro.2015.03.036.
7. Marti D, Spross C, Jost B. The first 100 elbow arthroscopies of one surgeon: analysis of complications. J Shoulder Elb Surg. 2013;22(4):567–73. https://doi.org/10.1016/j.jse.2012.12.001.
8. Savoie FH 3rd. Guidelines to becoming an expert elbow arthroscopist. Arthroscopy. 2007;23(11):1237–40. https://doi.org/10.1016/j.arthro.2007.04.013.
9. Werner BC, Fashandi AH, Chhabra AB, Deal DN. Effect of obesity on complication rate after elbow arthroscopy in a Medicare population. Arthroscopy. 2016;32(3):453–7. https://doi.org/10.1016/j.arthro.2015.08.025.
10. Babcock HM, Carroll C, Matava M, L'Ecuyer P, Fraser V. Surgical site infections after arthroscopy: outbreak investigation and case control study. Arthroscopy. 2003;19(2):172–81. https://doi.org/10.1053/jars.2003.50016.
11. Bert JM, Giannini D, Nace L. Antibiotic prophylaxis for arthroscopy of the knee: is it necessary? Arthroscopy. 2007;23(1):4–6. https://doi.org/10.1016/j.arthro.2006.08.014.
12. Muller-Rath R, Ingenhoven E, Mumme T, Schumacher M, Miltner O. Perioperatives Management in der ambulanten arthroskopischen Chirurgie des Kniegelenks. Z Orthop Unfall. 2010;148(3):282–7. https://doi.org/10.1055/s-0029-1240784.
13. Kurzweil PR. Antibiotic prophylaxis for arthroscopic surgery. Arthroscopy. 2006;22(4):452–4. https://doi.org/10.1016/j.arthro.2006.02.004.
14. AWMF. S1 Leitlinie "Perioperative Antibiotikaprophylaxe". 2012 [Zugegriffen 2018 Januar 24]. http://www.awmf.org/uploads/tx_szleitlinien/029-0221_S1_Perioperative_Antibiotikaprophylaxe_2012–02.pdf
15. Hauer T, Tabori E. Perioperative Antibiotikaprophylaxe (PAP). Arthroskopie. 2008;21(2):80–2. https://doi.org/10.1007/s00142-008-0444-4.
16. Reddy AS, Kvitne RS, Yocum LA, Elattrache NS, Glousman RE, Jobe FW. Arthroscopy of the elbow: a long-term clinical review. Arthroscopy. 2000;16(6):588–94. https://doi.org/10.1053/jars.2000.8953.
17. O'Driscoll SW, Morrey BF. Arthroscopy of the elbow. Diagnostic and therapeutic benefits and hazards. J Bone Joint Surg Am. 1992;74(1):84–94.
18. Morrey BF. Complications of elbow arthroscopy. Instr Course Lect. 2000;49:255–8.
19. Alexander JW, Solomkin JS, Edwards MJ. Updated recommendations for control of surgical site infections. Ann Surg. 2011;253(6):1082–93. https://doi.org/10.1097/SLA.0b013e31821175f8.
20. Reichman DE, Greenberg JA. Reducing surgical site infections: a review. Rev Obstet Gynecol. 2009;2(4):212–21. https://doi.org/10.3909/riog0084.
21. Kramer A, Assadian O, Gruber B, Lademann J. Prävention von postoperativen Wundinfektionen, Teil 1: Prä-operative Maßnahmen – Einfluss der Haarentfernung. Hyg Med. 2008;33(10):402–7.
22. Micheli LJ, Luke AC, Mintzer CM, Waters PM. Elbow arthroscopy in the pediatric and adolescent population. Arthroscopy. 2001;17(7):694–9. https://doi.org/10.1053/jars.2001.25338.
23. Müller-Rath R, Becker J, Ingenhoven E. Wie hoch ist das statistische Risiko einer Infektion nach ambulanter Arthroskopie? Arthroskopie. 2008;21(2):87–91. https://doi.org/10.1007/s00142-008-0445-3.
24. Jolley BJ, Martin HD, Miley G, Lee JAE. The effect of intra-articular steroid injection on arthroscopy infection rates. Arthroscopy. 1993;9(3):351.
25. Paul J, Kirchhoff C, Imhoff AB, Hinterwimmer S. Infektion nach Arthroskopie. Orthopade. 2008;37(11):1048–55. https://doi.org/10.1007/s00132-008-1309-2.

26. El Hajj F, Hoteit M, Ouaknine M. Elbow arthroscopy: an alternative to anteromedial portals. Orthop Traumatol Surg Res. 2015;101(4):411–4. https://doi.org/10.1016/j.otsr.2015.03.011.
27. Lynch GJ, Meyers JF, Whipple TL, Caspari RB. Neurovascular anatomy and elbow arthroscopy: inherent risks. Arthroscopy. 1986;2(3):190–7.
28. Schneider T, Hoffstetter I, Fink B, Jerosch J. Long-term results of elbow arthroscopy in 67 patients. Acta Orthop Belg. 1994;60(4):378–83.
29. Steinmann SP. Elbow arthroscopy: where are we now? Arthroscopy. 2007;23(11):1231–6. https://doi.org/10.1016/j.arthro.2007.08.008.
30. Desai MJ, Mithani SK, Lodha SJ, Richard MJ, Leversedge FJ, Ruch DS. Major peripheral nerve injuries after elbow arthroscopy. Arthroscopy. 2016;32:999–1002.e8. https://doi.org/10.1016/j.arthro.2015.11.023.
31. Elfeddali R, Schreuder MH, Eygendaal D. Arthroscopic elbow surgery, is it safe? J Shoulder Elb Surg. 2013;22(5):647–52. https://doi.org/10.1016/j.jse.2013.01.032.
32. Ruch DS, Poehling GG. Anterior interosseous nerve injury following elbow arthroscopy. Arthroscopy. 1997;13(6):756–8.
33. Abboud JA, Ricchetti ET, Tjoumakaris F, Ramsey ML. Elbow arthroscopy: basic setup and portal placement. J Am Acad Orthop Surg. 2006;14(5):312–8.
34. Gallay SH, Richards RR, O'Driscoll SW. Intraarticular capacity and compliance of stiff and normal elbows. Arthroscopy. 1993;9(1):9–13.
35. Adolfsson L. Arthroscopy of the elbow joint: a cadaveric study of portal placement. J Shoulder Elb Surg. 1994;3(2):53–61. https://doi.org/10.1016/S1058-2746(09)80110-9.
36. Drescher H, Schwering L, Jerisch J, Herzig M. The risk of neurovascular damage in elbow joint arthroscopy. Which approach is better: anteromedial or anterolateral? Z Orthop Ihre Grenzgeb. 1994;132(2):120–5.
37. Field LD, Altchek DW, Warren RF, O'Brien SJ, Skyhar MJ, Wickiewicz TL. Arthroscopic anatomy of the lateral elbow: a comparison of three portals. Arthroscopy. 1994;10(6):602–7.
38. Imhoff AB, Feucht M. Atlas sportorthopädisch-sporttraumatologische Operationen. Berlin, Heidelberg: Springer; 2017.
39. Park JY, Cho CH, Choi JH, Lee ST, Kang CH. Radial nerve palsy after arthroscopic anterior capsular release for degenerative elbow contracture. Arthroscopy. 2007;23(12):1360.e1–3. https://doi.org/10.1016/j.arthro.2006.11.021.
40. Haapaniemi T, Berggren M, Adolfsson L. Complete transection of the median and radial nerves during arthroscopic release of post-traumatic elbow contracture. Arthroscopy. 1999;15(7):784–7.
41. Hackl M, Lappen S, Burkhart KJ, et al. Elbow positioning and joint insufflation substantially influence median and radial nerve locations. Clin Orthop Relat Res. 2015;473(11):3627–34. https://doi.org/10.1007/s11999-015-4442-3.
42. Miller CD, Jobe CM, Wright MH. Neuroanatomy in elbow arthroscopy. J Shoulder Elb Surg. 1995;4(3):168–74.
43. Lüring C, Tingart M. Operative Zugangswege in Orthopädie und Unfallchirurgie. Berlin, Heidelberg: Springer; 2015.
44. Omid R, Hamid N, Keener JD, Galatz LM, Yamaguchi K. Relation of the radial nerve to the anterior capsule of the elbow: anatomy with correlation to arthroscopy. Arthroscopy. 2012;28(12):1800–4. https://doi.org/10.1016/j.arthro.2012.05.890.
45. Unlu MC, Kesmezacar H, Akgun I, Ogut T, Uzun I. Anatomic relationship between elbow arthroscopy portals and neurovascular structures in different elbow and forearm positions. J Shoulder Elb Surg. 2006;15(4):457–62. https://doi.org/10.1016/j.jse.2005.09.012.
46. Gay DM, Raphael BS, Weiland AJ. Revision arthroscopic contracture release in the elbow resulting in an ulnar nerve transection: a case report. J Bone Joint Surg Am. 2010;92(5):1246–9. https://doi.org/10.2106/JBJS.I.00555.
47. Hahn M, Grossmann JA. Ulnar nerve laceration as a result of elbow arthroscopy. J Hand Surg Br. 1998;23(1):109.
48. Huffman GR, O'Driscoll SW. Delayed onset ulnar neuropathy after arthroscopic elbow contracture release (SS-63). Arthroscopy. 2006;22(6):e32. https://doi.org/10.1016/j.arthro.2006.04.065.
49. Blonna D, O'Driscoll SW. Delayed-onset ulnar neuritis after release of elbow contracture: preventive strategies derived from a study of 563 cases. Arthroscopy. 2014;30(8):947–56. https://doi.org/10.1016/j.arthro.2014.03.022.
50. Sahajpal DT, Blonna D, O'Driscoll SW. Anteromedial elbow arthroscopy portals in patients with prior ulnar nerve transposition or subluxation. Arthroscopy. 2010;26(8):1045–52. https://doi.org/10.1016/j.arthro.2009.12.029.
51. Jupiter JB, O'Driscoll SW, Cohen MS. The assessment and management of the stiff elbow. Instr Course Lect. 2003;52:93–111.
52. Werner CM, Zimmermann SM, Wurgler-Hauri CC, Lane JM, Wanner GA, Simmen HP. Use of imatinib in the prevention of heterotopic ossification. HSS J. 2013;9(2):166–70. https://doi.org/10.1007/s11420-013-9335-y.
53. Zeckey C, Hildebrand F, Frink M, Krettek C. Heterotopic ossifications following implant surgery--epidemiology, therapeutical approaches and current concepts. Semin Immunopathol. 2011;33(3):273–86. https://doi.org/10.1007/s00281-011-0240-5.
54. Hastings H, Graham TJ. The classification and treatment of heterotopic ossification about the elbow and forearm. Hand Clin. 1994;10(3):417–37.
55. Gofton WT, King GJ. Heterotopic ossification following elbow arthroscopy. Arthroscopy. 2001;17(1):E2. https://doi.org/10.1053/jars.2001.16283.

56. Hughes SC, Hildebrand KA. Heterotopic ossification--a complication of elbow arthroscopy: a case report. J Shoulder Elb Surg. 2010;19(1):e1–5. https://doi.org/10.1016/j.jse.2009.04.015.
57. Sodha S, Nagda SH, Sennett BJ. Heterotopic ossification in a throwing athlete after elbow arthroscopy. Arthroscopy. 2006;22(7):802.e1–3. https://doi.org/10.1016/j.arthro.2005.05.035.
58. Kölbl O, Barthel T, Krödel A, Seegen-Schmiedt MH. Prevention of heterotopic ossification after hip arthroplastys. Dtsch Arztebl. 2003;100(45):2441–9.
59. Salazar D, Golz A, Israel H, Marra G. Heterotopic ossification of the elbow treated with surgical resection: risk factors, bony ankylosis, and complications. Clin Orthop Relat Res. 2014;472(7):2269–75. https://doi.org/10.1007/s11999-014-3591-0.
60. Amstutz HC, Fowble VA, Schmalzried TP, Dorey FJ. Short-course indomethacin prevents heterotopic ossification in a high-risk population following total hip arthroplasty. J Arthroplast. 1997;12(2):126–32.
61. Eulert J, Knelles D, Barthel T. Heterotope Ossifikationen. Unfallchirurg. 1997;100(8):667–74.
62. Neal BC, Rodgers A, Clark T, et al. A systematic survey of 13 randomized trials of non-steroidal anti-inflammatory drugs for the prevention of heterotopic bone formation after major hip surgery. Acta Orthop Scand. 2000;71(2):122–8. https://doi.org/10.1080/000164700317413076.
63. Rivera JC, Hsu JR, Noel SP, Wenke JC, Rathbone CR. Locally delivered nonsteroidal anti-inflammatory drug: a potential option for heterotopic ossification prevention. Clin Transl Sci. 2015;8(5):591–3. https://doi.org/10.1111/cts.12300.
64. Abrams RA, Simmons BP, Brown RA, Botte MJ. Treatment of posttraumatic radioulnar synostosis with excision and low dose radiation. J Hand Surg Am. 1993;18(4):703–7. https://doi.org/10.1016/0363-5023(93)90322-T.
65. McAuliffe JA, Wolfson AH. Early excision of heterotopic ossification about the elbow followed by radiation therapy. J Bone Joint Surg Am. 1997;79(5):749–55.
66. Robinson CG, Polster JM, Reddy CA, et al. Postoperative single-fraction radiation for prevention of heterotopic ossification of the elbow. Int J Radiat Oncol Biol Phys. 2010;77(5):1493–9. https://doi.org/10.1016/j.ijrobp.2009.06.072.
67. Evans PJ, Nandi S, Maschke S, Hoyen HA, Lawton JN. Prevention and treatment of elbow stiffness. J Hand Surg Am. 2009;34(4):769–78. https://doi.org/10.1016/j.jhsa.2009.02.020.
68. Garland DE. A clinical perspective on common forms of acquired heterotopic ossification. Clin Orthop Relat Res. 1991;263:13–29.
69. Viola RW, Hastings H 2nd. Treatment of ectopic ossification about the elbow. Clin Orthop Relat Res. 2000;(370):65–86.
70. Jupiter JB, Ring D. Operative treatment of post-traumatic proximal radioulnar synostosis. J Bone Joint Surg Am. 1998;80(2):248–57.
71. Moritomo H, Tada K, Yoshida T. Early, wide excision of heterotopic ossification in the medial elbow. J Shoulder Elb Surg. 2001;10(2):164–8. https://doi.org/10.1067/mse.2001.112055.
72. Tsionos I, Leclercq C, Rochet JM. Heterotopic ossification of the elbow in patients with burns. Results after early excision. J Bone Joint Surg Br. 2004;86(3):396–403. https://doi.org/10.1302/0301-620X.86B3.
73. Savoie FH, 3rd, O'Brien MJ, Wert M (2016) Early arthroscopic management of heterotopic ossification of the elbow. In: Savoie FH, 3rd, Field LD, Steinmann SP (eds) The elbow and wrist: AANA advanced arthroscopic surgical techniques. CRC Press
74. Wert M, Savoie FH 3rd. Early arthroscopic management strategies for patients developing moderate to severe heterotopic ossification of the elbow. Arthroscopy. 2013;29(6):e21. https://doi.org/10.1016/j.arthro.2013.03.050.
75. Grand JG, Roig JA, de Swarte M. Instrument breakage as a complication of elbow arthroscopy in a dog. Aust Vet J. 2014;92(4):128–31. https://doi.org/10.1111/avj.12153.
76. Thomas RJ, Savoie FH 3rd, Field LD. Complications of elbow arthroscopy (SS-67). Arthroscopy. 2007;23(6):e34. https://doi.org/10.1016/j.arthro.2007.03.081.
77. Fitzgibbons PG, Digiovanni C, Hares S, Akelman E. Safe tourniquet use: a review of the evidence. J Am Acad Orthop Surg. 2012;20(5):310–9. https://doi.org/10.5435/JAAOS-20-05-310.

Glossary

aMCL Anterior bundle of the medial collateral ligament (Chap. 4)

Anterolateral portal 1–2 cm anterior and 2 cm proximal to the lateral humeral epicondyle (Chap. 3)

Anteromedial portal 1–2 cm anterior and 2 cm proximal to the medial humeral epicondyle (Chap. 3)

Arthrofibrosis, post-traumatic 3 months after trauma, signs of stagnation, tendency to improve after 12 months (Chap. 9)

Bare area Cartilage-free area of the trochlea (trochlear notch) (Chap. 1)

Broberg-Morrey score Score (max. 100 points (points): 40 points mobility, 20 points strength, 5 points stability, 35 points pain)

CEO Common extensor origin (Chap. 7)

Chondromatosis Rare cartilage-forming metaplasia of the synovium, risk of secondary osteoarthritis and rarely degeneration into chondrosarcoma (Chap. 5)

Coronoid process Ventral hook-shaped process of the olecranon; most important osseous AP and varus stabilizer (Chap. 1)

CRAP Classification system for lateral elbow pain (Chap. 7)

CRPS Complex regional pain syndrome (Chap. 9)

Dubberley classification Classification of shear fractures of the capitulum (Chap. 11)

ECRB Extensor carpi radialis brevis (Chap. 7)

Fat Pad Sign Radiological indication of "bleeding in the joint" (Chap. 1)

Functional ROM 0–30–100° range of motion (Chap. 1)

Graham and Hastings classification Four-stage development of heterotopic ossification (Chap. 10)

High posterolateral portal 1–2 cm proximal to the tip of the olecranon on the edge of the triceps tendon (Chap. 3)

Incisura radialis (radial notch) Ulnar part of the proximal radio-ulnar joint (PRUG), resection plane for resection of the radial head (Chap. 1)

Inflow cannula Mostly inserted through the anterolateral portal (Chap. 3)

Interosseous membrane Connecting the radius and ulna, load/force transfer from radial distal to ulnar proximal (Chap. 1)

Kay classification of elbow stiffness Soft tissue contraction without ossification—fracture without dislocation—post-traumatic bony blockages (Chap. 9)

LCL Lateral collateral ligament (Chap. 1)

LUCL Lateral ulnar collateral ligament (Chap. 1)

MACT Matrix-induced autologous cartilage cell transplantation (Chap. 4)

Mason classification (1–4) (Chap. 11)

Morrey classification of elbow stiffness Combined extrinsically and intrinsically (Chap. 9)

MUCL Medial ulnar collateral ligament (Chap. 1)

O'Driscoll classification CT classification of the coronoid fractures taking into account the three-dimensional size (Chap. 6)

OATS Osteochondral autologous transplant system

A. B. Imhoff, A. Lenich (eds.), *Elbow Arthroscopy and Minimal Invasive Surgery*,
https://doi.org/10.1007/978-3-031-75611-5

OCL Osteochondral lesion due to microtraumas (Chap. 4)

Osborne-Cotterill lesion Osteochondral lesion of the dorsal capitulum with avulsion of the lateral ulnar collateral ligament (LUCL)—"Bankart lesion" of the elbow (Chap. 1)

Osborn arcade Connection between the medial humeral epicondyle and the flexor carpi ulnaris muscle (distal constriction of the ulnar nerve) (Chap. 1)

Osteochondral shear test Moving the elbow with closed fist: crepitation positive (Chap. 4)

Osteochondritis dissecans (OD) Aseptic, mostly traumatic bone necrosis of a circumscribed articular surface area (Chap. 4)

Panner's disease Juvenile osteonecrosis of the capitulum (Chap. 4)

PIN Posterior interosseous nerve of the radial nerve, innervates extensors of the forearm (Chap. 11)

PLRI Posterolateral rotational instability (Chap. 7)

Posterocentral portal syn.: transtricipital; 3–4 cm proximal to the tip of the olecranon through the triceps tendon (Chap. 3)

Proximal anterolateral/anteromedial portals Accessory portals located approx. 1 cm proximal to the corresponding standard portal (Chap. 3)

PRUJ Proximal radioulnar joint (Chap. 1)

Radial bow 17–18° radial angulation of the proximal ulna (Chap. 1)

Radius head angle 22 mm diameter, radius head-neck angle 10–12° (Chap. 1)

Regan-Morrey classification of coronoid fractures Based on the fragment size in the lateral X-ray view, comparable to O'Driscoll classification (Chap. 11)

Soft spot (= deep dorsoradial) portal Dorsoradially in the center between the radial head, olecranon, and lateral epicondyle (Chap. 3)

Steroid infiltration Both preoperatively and intraoperatively procedure that increases the risk of complications (Chap. 13)

Struthers arcade Passage of the ulnar nerve at the medial intermuscular septum (proximal) (Chap. 1)

Subliminal tuberosity Anteromedial facet of the coronoid, insertion of the anterior bundle of the medial collateral ligament (aMCL) (Chap. 1)

Supracondylar process Atavistic protrusion 6–7 cm proximal to the joint space on the ventroulnar humerus (Chap. 1)

Valgus angle/support angle 6–8° valgus angle physiologically (Chap. 1)

FSC
www.fsc.org
MIX
Papier aus verantwortungsvollen Quellen
Paper from responsible sources
FSC® C105338

If you have any concerns about our products,
you can contact us on
ProductSafety@springernature.com

In case Publisher is established outside the EU,
the EU authorized representative is:
Springer Nature Customer Service Center GmbH
Europaplatz 3, 69115 Heidelberg, Germany

Printed by Libri Plureos GmbH
in Hamburg, Germany